Jay Kordich's
Live Foods Live Bodies!

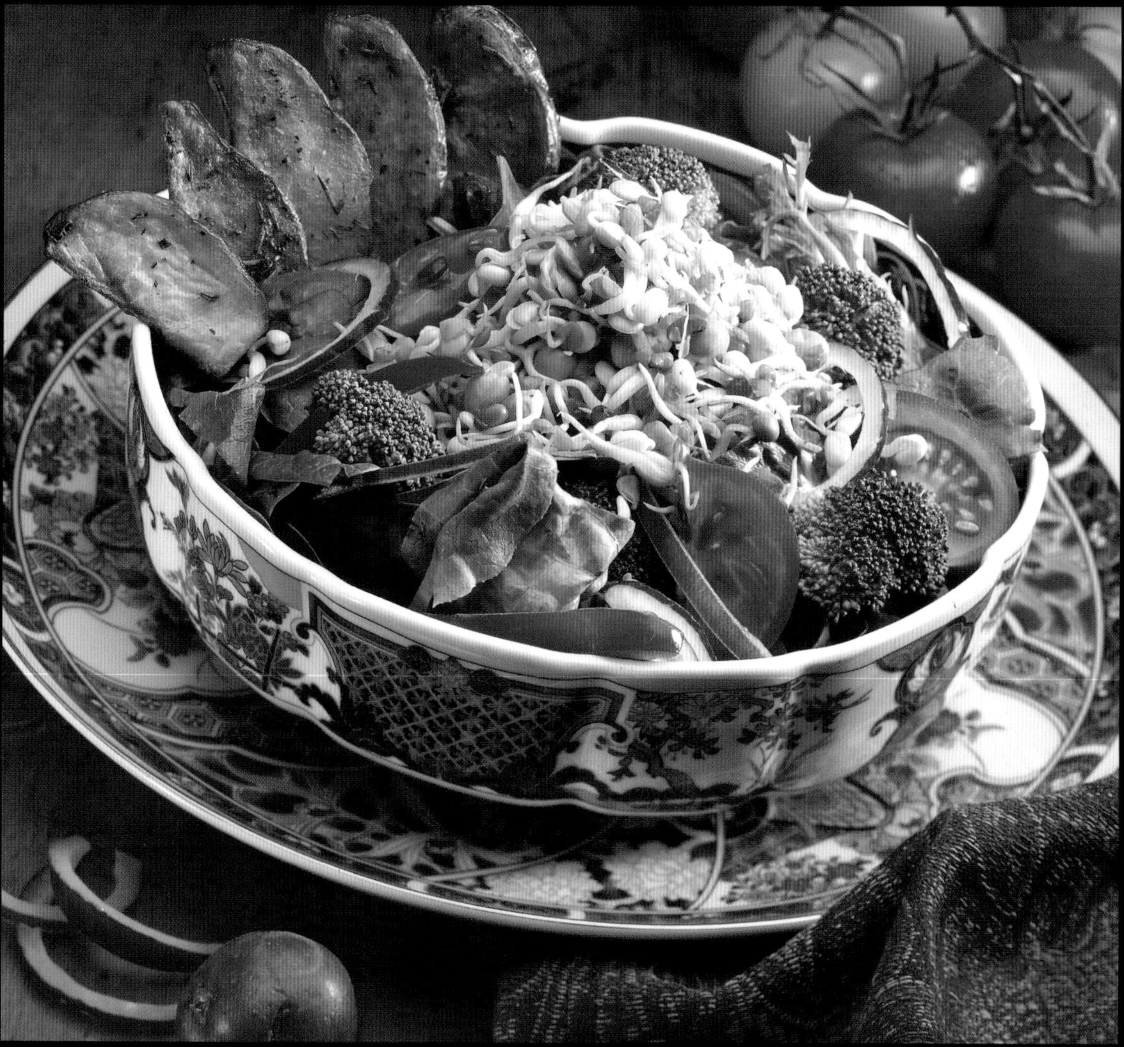

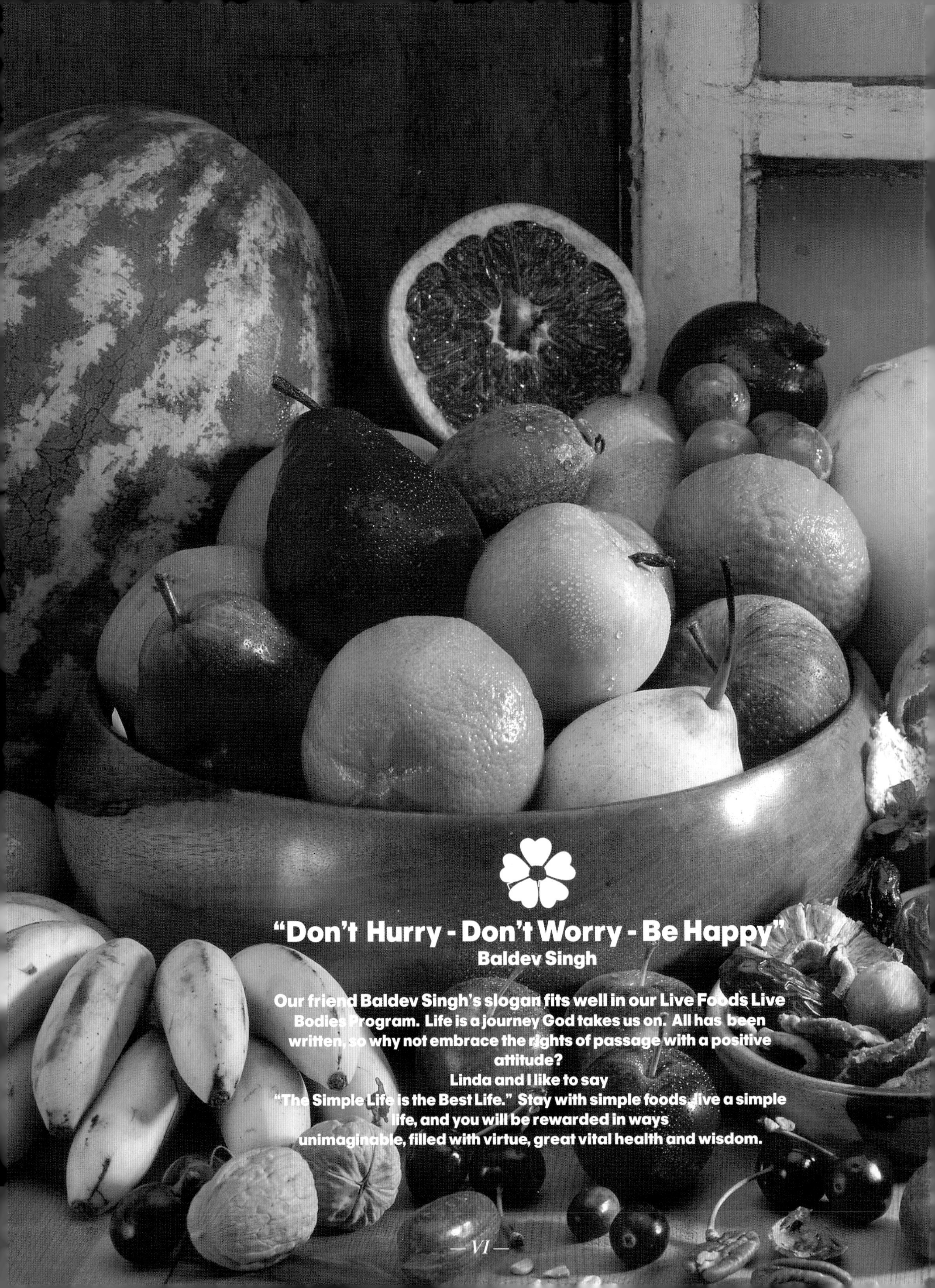

“Don’t Hurry - Don’t Worry - Be Happy”

Baldev Singh

Our friend Baldev Singh’s slogan fits well in our Live Foods Live Bodies Program. Life is a journey God takes us on. All has been written, so why not embrace the rights of passage with a positive attitude?

Linda and I like to say
“The Simple Life is the Best Life.” Stay with simple foods, live a simple life, and you will be rewarded in ways unimaginable, filled with virtue, great vital health and wisdom.

Live Foods Live Bodies!

"We make Food come Alive"

Jay and Linda Kordich

Kordich House Press

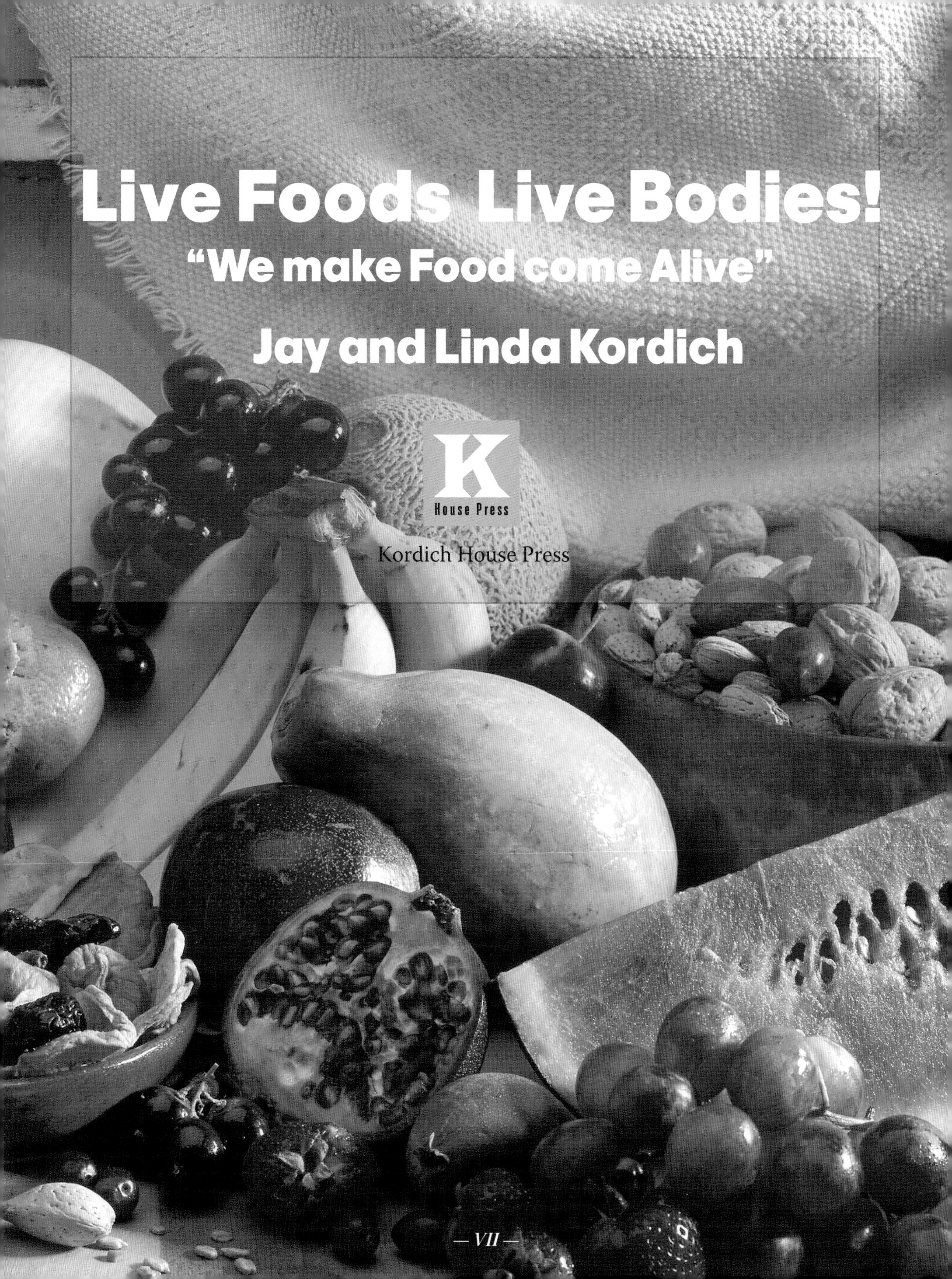

Our Loving Dedication

***This book** is lovingly dedicated to our beloved children, the only family we have left in the world. Jayson and John, we aspire to share all that we know with others because of the stellar love and dedication you lovingly give to us. We dedicate this book to you and to Cheryl, as you have so beautifully and joyfully inspired our lives to be greater than it could ever be.*

We hold this book near and dear to our hearts knowing that you have helped us to make this dream a reality. When there didn't seem to be any faith, you had it to give, with patience and inspiration to believe we could continue when we thought all was lost and gone is a demonstration and validation of just how great you truly are.

Matt Becker and Donna Jensen, without your unconditional love, where would we be? We feel rich inside knowing you are our true friends.

We also dedicate this book to you, the reader. You, who have the courage to change for the better, to see there is indeed a new you waiting to be born. Share this knowledge with those you love and with those who are in need. Illness and degenerative disease does not have to be in our future. Millions of people die every year of diseases we believe are reversible through diet and lifestyle.

Aspire to live the real-life dream of vital health, longevity and super awareness faithfully waiting for you!

Jay and Linda Kordich

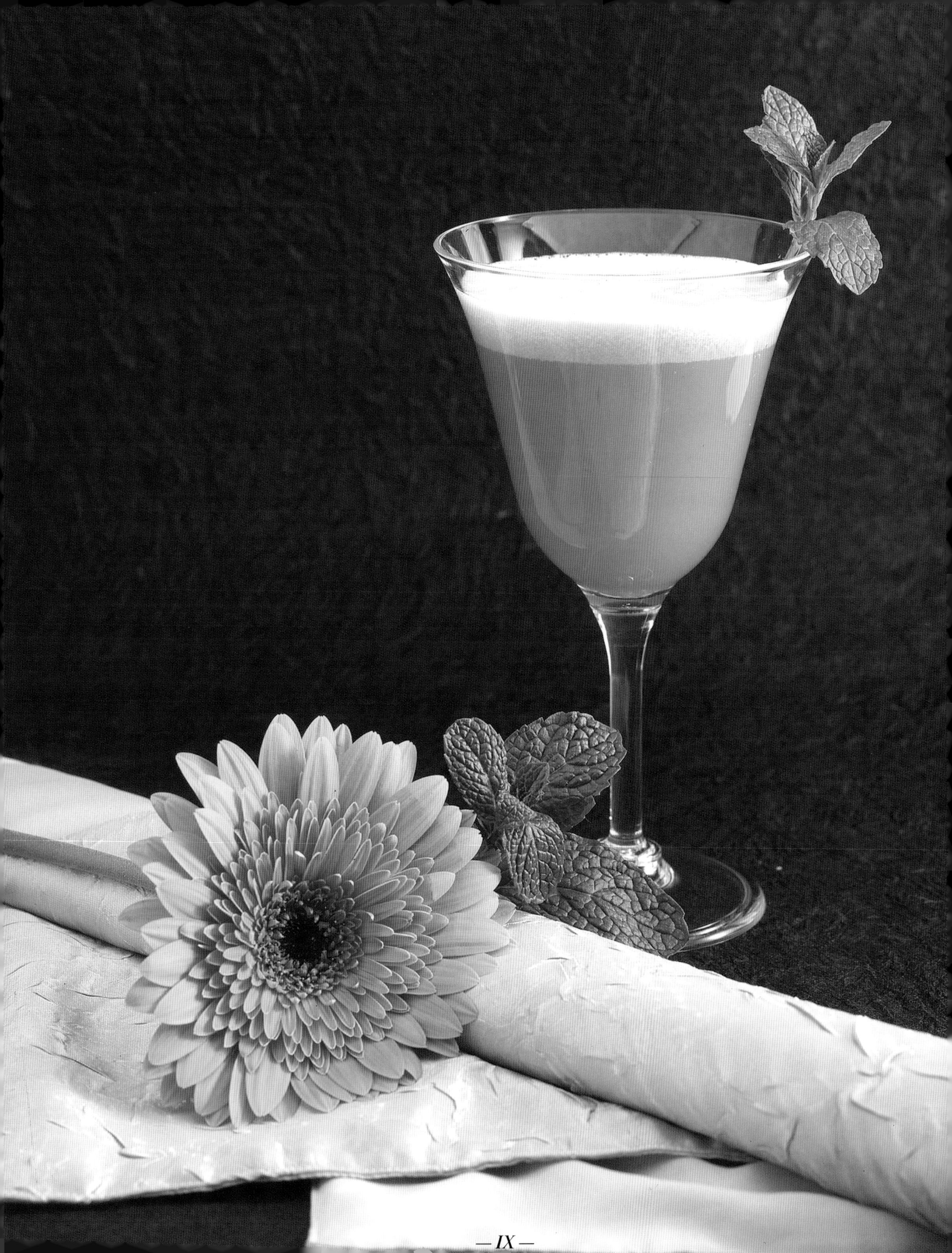

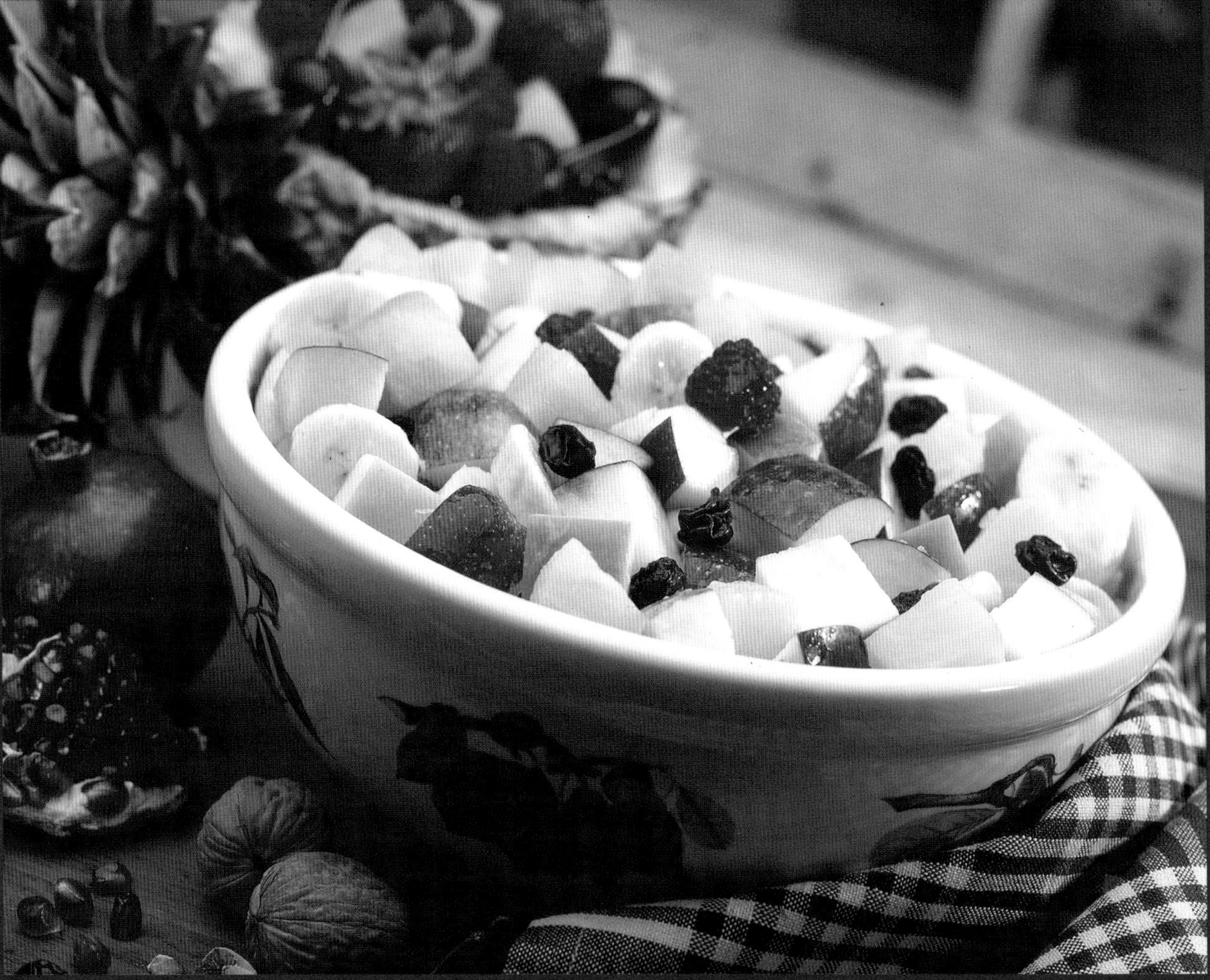

For more information on getting permission for reprints and/or excerpts, please contact:
Kordich Group International, Inc.
PO Box 3486
Rancho Santa Fe, CA 92067

Find us on the web at:
www.jaykordich.com

Live Foods Live Bodies is a registered trademark of Kordich Group International, Inc.
ISBN 0-9749212-0-3

Printed and bound in China by Kaleido Graphic Services Group, Inc.

Photo credits: Edmond Fong, Cheryl Tsai, Linda Kordich, Ben Ged Low

Book Design: Cheryl Tsai and Linda Kordich

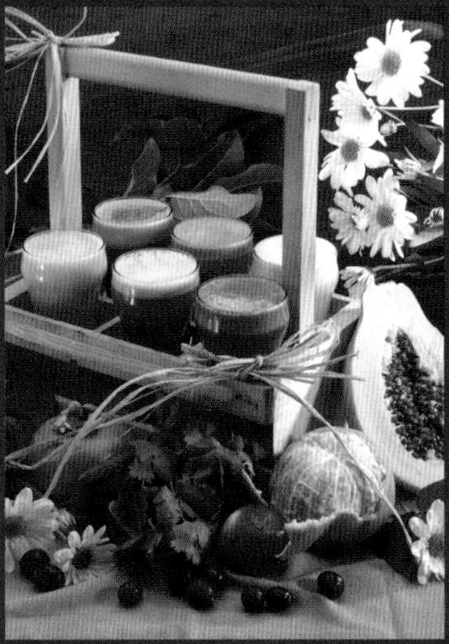

Part I

Chapter 1 Starting Over 4-7

Chapter 2 The Power of Juicing 10-23

Chapter 3 Color Me Green 26-41

Chapter 4 Enzymes = Energy 44-51

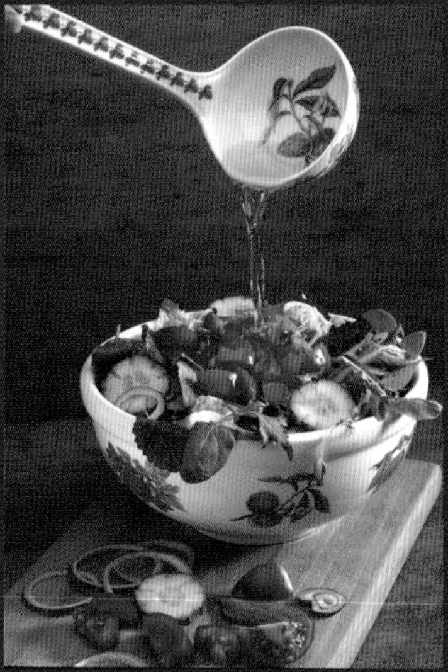

Part II

Chapter 5 The Power of Living Foods 56-71

Chapter 6 Our Living Kitchen 74-87

Chapter 7 The Art of The Salad 90-105

Chapter 8 - Our Living Recipes 108-217

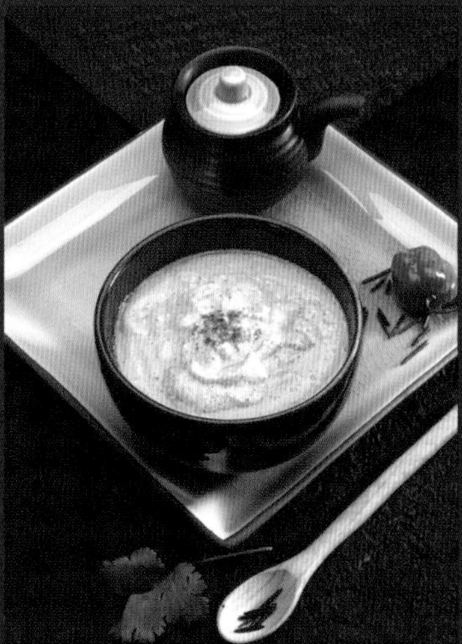

Our Websites and Resources 220-225

Index 228-233

"When you Have
you Have a Futu

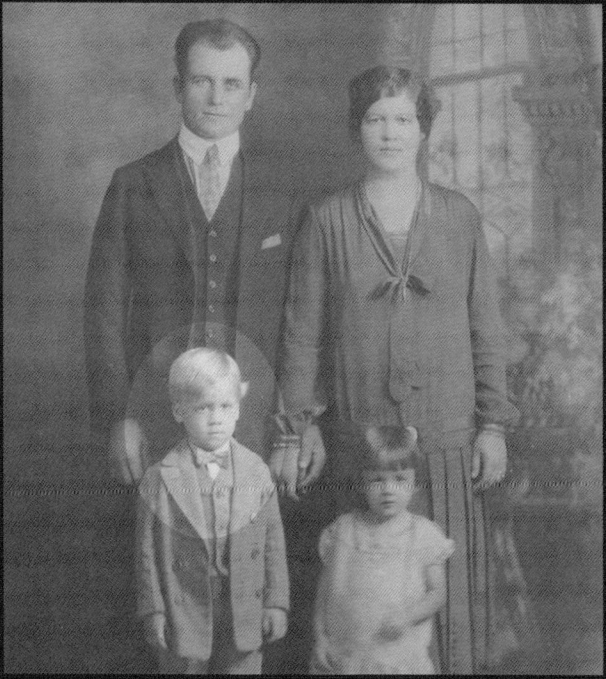

Family photo of Me, My Sister and My Parents in 1926

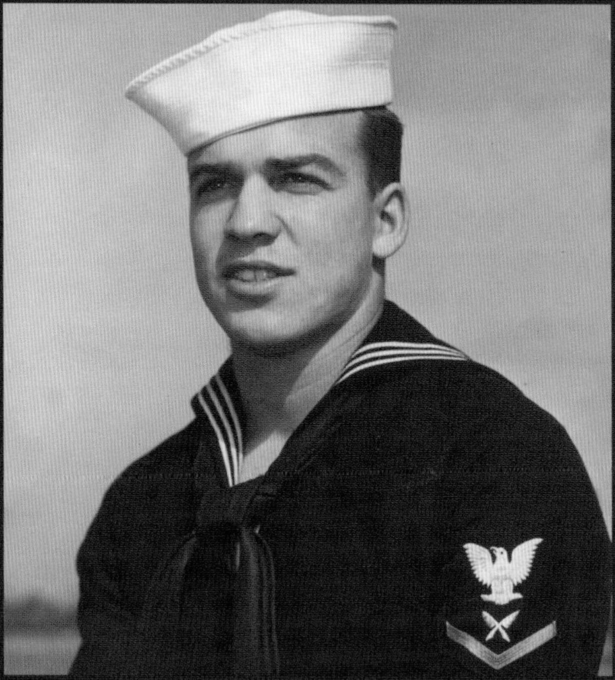

Here I am serving in the Navy in World War II

your Health
re" – Jay Kordich

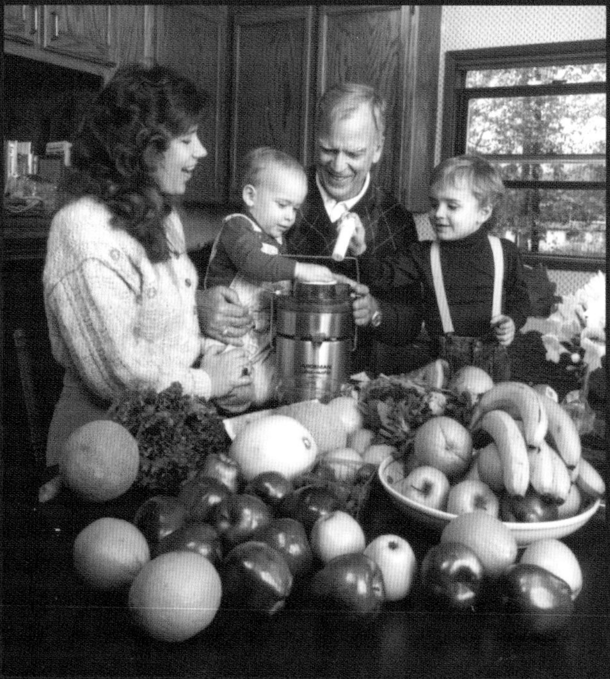

My wife Linda, John, Jayson and Me in 1987

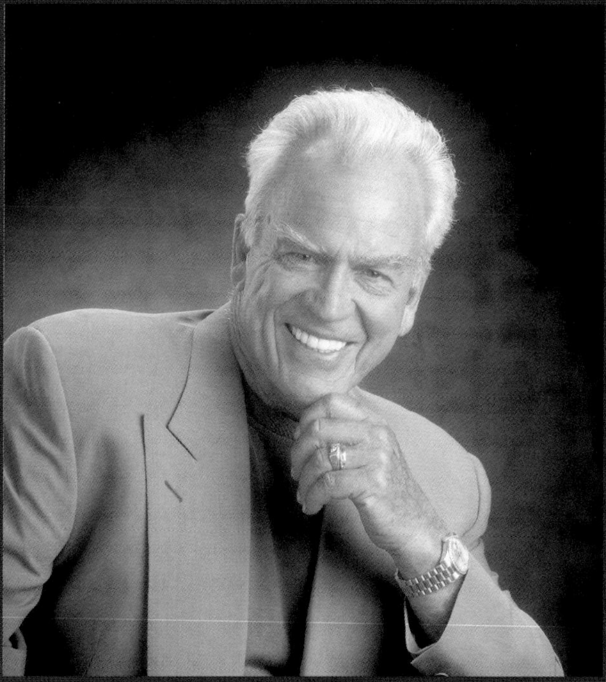

Here I am in my 80s!

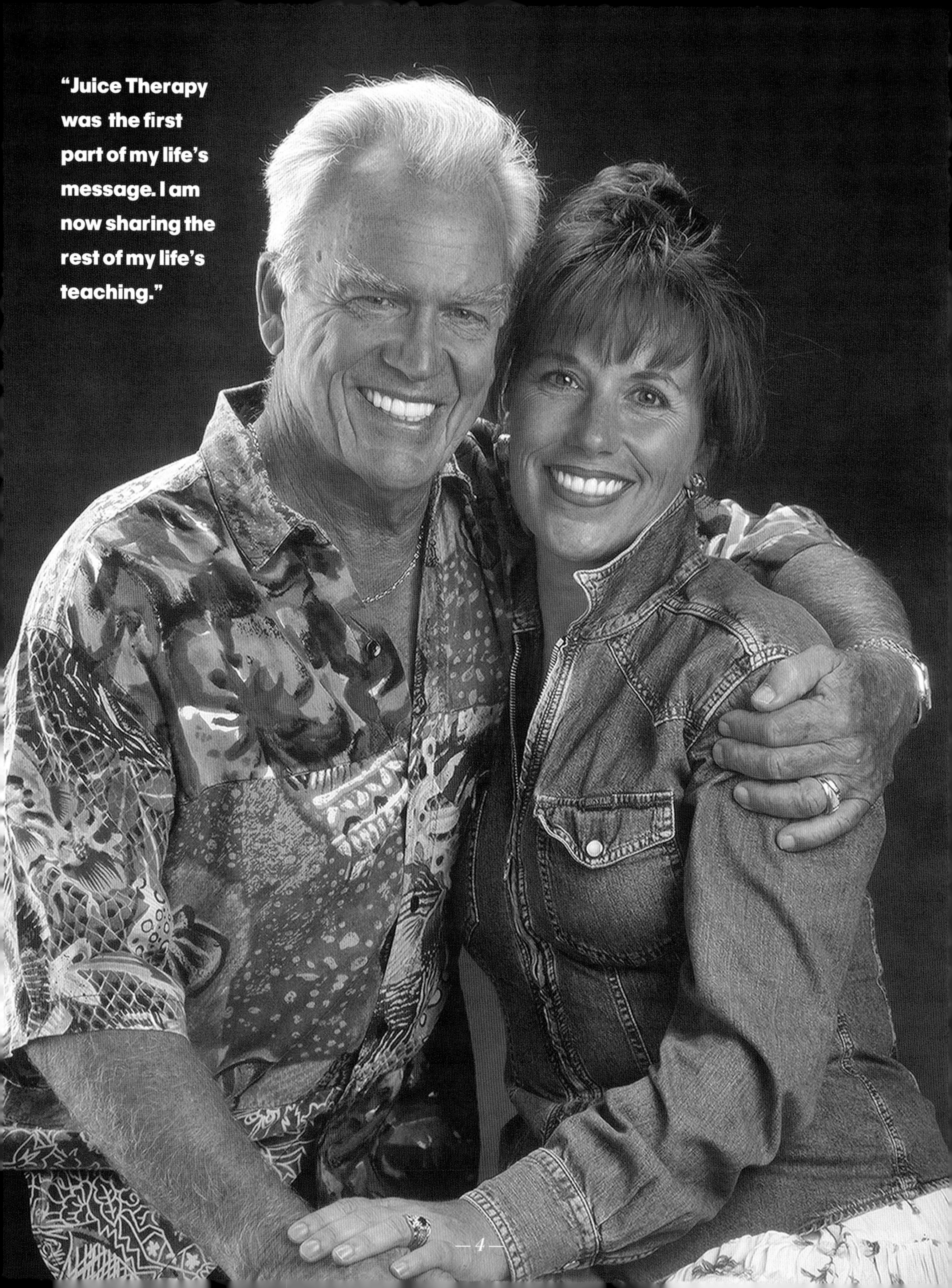
"Juice Therapy was the first part of my life's message. I am now sharing the rest of my life's teaching."

Chapter 1

Starting Over

What you have in your hands is the power to change your life. Live Foods Live Bodies is truly a revolutionary program my wife, Linda, and I have practiced collectively for close to 90 years—for fifty-seven years of my life and twenty-five years of Linda's. Because we have dedicated our entire adult lives to the highest standards of living health, you can be assured that Linda and I are experts in our field and can offer you solid guidance in attaining your own vital health and longevity.

Do you remember Me?....

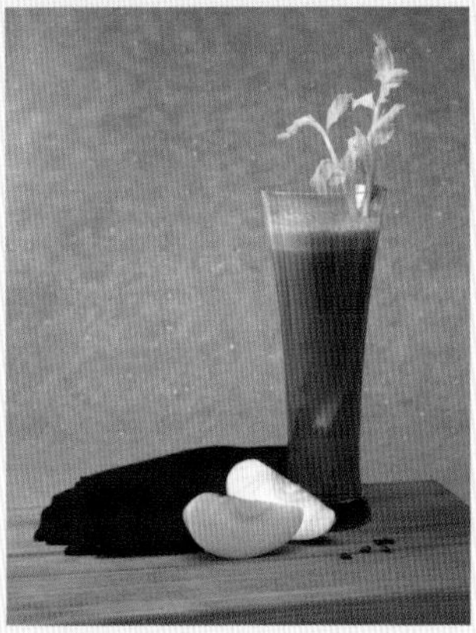

You may remember me from my #1 book on The New York Times Best-selling list: The Power of Juicing. What you may not know is that I have been retired for quite some time. Unfortunately, back in 1998, I lost the right to use my trademark name I've become so well known as. Due to this restriction, Linda and I have not been able to reach the public to teach this message because many publishers do not want to take the risk to publish under my own name, Jay Kordich. However, it's very important to me to be able to share the rest of our story about how you can attain vital health, everyday.

So, back in 2001, Linda and I decided to make lemonade out of lemons and become publishers ourselves. Now we can reach you directly, through our own publishing company, *Kordich House Press.*

As I like to say, juice therapy was the first part of my message. Juicing is not just about putting fruits together that taste good. In this book you will find some of the best healing juice therapy recipes I have been using for the past 57 years.

Perhaps you have seen my infomercial in which I've sold the Juicer and taught millions of Americans about the life-giving benefits of fresh juicing. However, juicing is only the first part of my life's message. I am now sharing my life's teaching, this time, through a multi-media program that took us more than three years to create and gives you the same understanding it has taken Linda and me decades to develop.

Our best advice is to take it slow, read each chapter and transition your new lifestyle without beating yourself up if you slip every now and then. Slow and steady wins the race.

Buying a Juicer is just the Beginning

We hope to help you recognize that buying health-promoting appliances, juicers included, is a great start. But if they sit unused in your kitchen, they offer you no value. Enthusiastic and regular use of appliances like a juicer comes from the knowledge and application we offer you now. Inspiration combined with applied knowledge is the *KEY* to success in any venture. Our quick and easy-to-follow system provides you with the necessary understanding, motivation, and integration that will transform your limited perception of what "real vital health" is, into a lifelong appreciation and, most importantly, knowing how to take action.

This is where the real *"juice"* of the teaching begins. Trust me; juicing has been my life's teaching and savior for almost sixty years. I have also spent my entire adult life teaching about the power behind living foods and enzymes, which I now share with you in this book. It's our belief we really can live disease free lives way into our nineties, with all our faculties in good order.

The Strength behind Me

My original juicing message on television was launched successfully, to the expertise of Linda. She is the strength behind all that I do. She and I have lived an empowering juicing and eating lifestyle during our twenty-five years of marriage. In fact, Linda became a vegetarian when she was ten years old, back in 1965, and was an advocate of juicing long before we met. While I was known as that 'Juiceguy', Linda is known as an expert in her own right as a vegetarian/vegan teacher and living-foods proponent. Together, not only do we make a knowledgeable and experienced team, but we make the most delicious and satisfying foods and juices, ever!

When you begin this program, you'll feel as if you're eating with Linda and me. While my focus has seemingly been only on juicing, the message has always been the same: *Live Foods Live Bodies.* Linda and I now invite you to hear the rest of our story—the story of how you can create like we did, your own Living Kitchen, and how to incorporate and integrate vitality to your health, stamina, and a long, disease-free life for yourself and your family. The greatest gift I can give you before I leave this world is to teach you these priceless principles of living health that have worked successfully for me for over 57 years

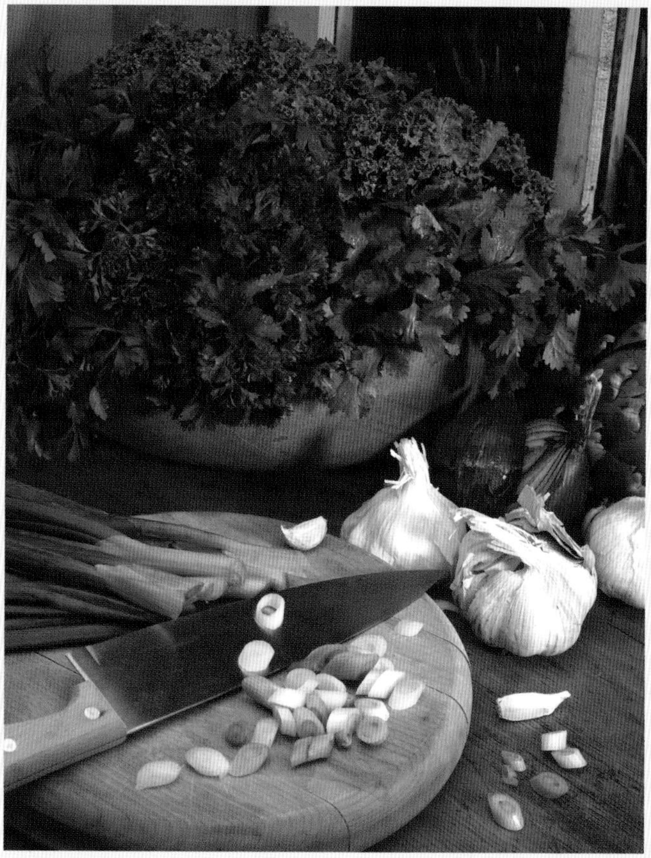

Doing it our Way is Easy

Living foods are powerful, whether in juice or food form. Our bodies need live, fresh, colorful fruits and vegetables full of enzymes, the catalysts of vitality to be ingested every single day. This can be a daunting venture, but just wait. You will begin to see it's not hard at all. You are going to learn a lot about enzymes when you read this book. Enzymes are the missing link to longevity and disease-free living. Back in the 1940's, '50's, '60's '70's, '80's, and part of the '90's, I used to call the properties of fresh juices the *"yet unidentified"* elements of life and growth. Now scientists and researchers have identified them as phyto-nutrients, which means plant nutrients. Fresh juices are filled with these phyto-nutrients and enzymes, the actual vital forces behind disease-free living.

Living Foods =Flavor!

Most people used to think vegetable juices were boring and tasteless. Some people once thought carrot juice was strange, yet when they met me and tasted my juice combinations, most never dreamed that carrot juice combined with apple could become an entirely new taste experience. It's the same with our Live Foods Live Bodies Program. Vegetarian foods have a reputation of being tasteless and boring, but when you have experts like Linda and me, you will discover it's the dressings, combinations, and spices that can literally change this old way of thinking. This program is so easy and enlightening that most people leave behind their old ways of eating without even realizing they've changed.

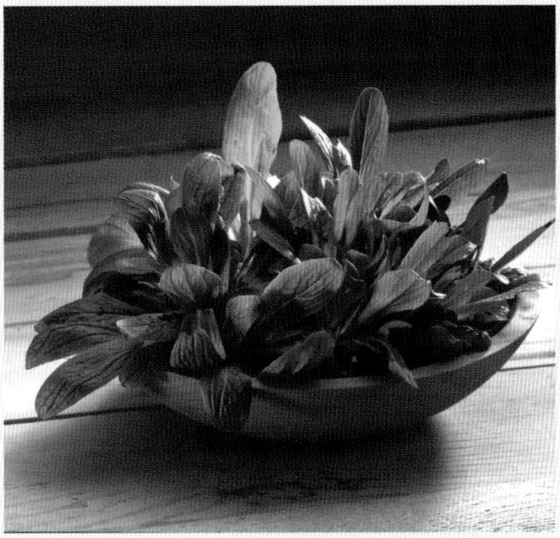

My Fall from Health

Close to sixty years ago, I was like most people, eating rich meats, dairy, sugar, and junk foods, not paying any attention to my health. But my body told me I had to shape up.

I was diagnosed with bladder cancer back in 1948 and was told I had less than one year to live. Luckily, I was both young and blessed with an open mind. I instinctively turned to nature and luckily found a well-known holistic cancer doctor from Germany, Dr. Max Gerson. He started me on a (raw) living foods and juice diet that would change my life forever. Within 90 days I added some living foods and some cooked broths back into my diet, but this time, with a new awareness of how and when to eat them

Your Life will Change

Now at 82, I feel great. It is my passion and goal to share with everybody how it is possible to awake every morning to feel refreshed and not to face fatigue throughout the day. It is possible to live disease-free, full of stamina and vitality. It's never too late to regenerate our bodies. You wouldn't believe the stories we have heard. When people start juicing and paying attention to a more "raw" and living foods diet, they report that their aches and pains start to fall away. Their bowel and skin problems clear up. They report they have energy like they did when they were young.

Are you Ready?

Now, as you join us toward this new pathway of eating and living, you are about to learn my priceless secrets that have sustained me so long for all these years. The main secret I will reveal in this book is something I would like you to ask yourself every time you sit down to eat a meal: *How Much of my Meal is Living?* I know it sounds strange at first, but, believe me, when you are finished with this book, you will understand what this really means. I cover this in detail in Chapter 5. By understanding what living foods really are, this simple awareness will be the key to ultimately transforming the way you eat forever.

If you want to start over in life, needing a new direction and change, just remember this: *If I can start over at the age of eighty-two, indeed you can too.* What we all need is a support system and trust in someone who has traveled these roads before, as we have.

Our Personal Resources on page 228, can really help.

"It's the Juice that Feeds You

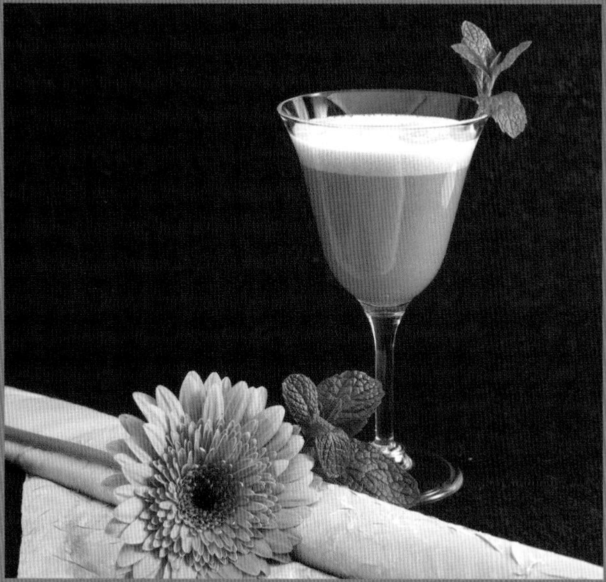

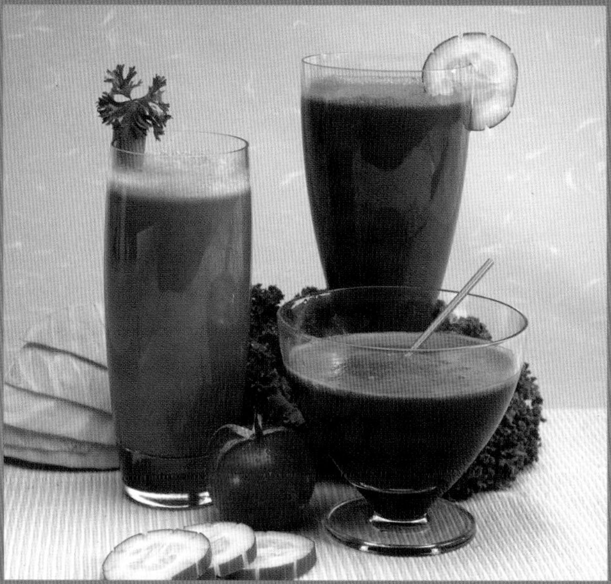

of the Fiber

’ - *Jay Kordich*

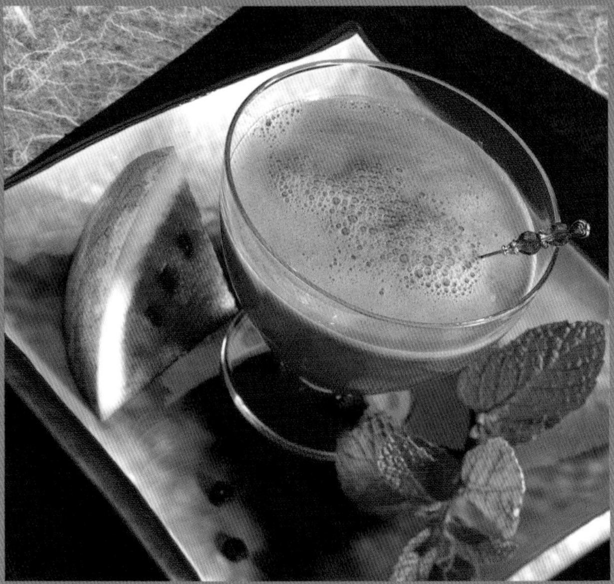

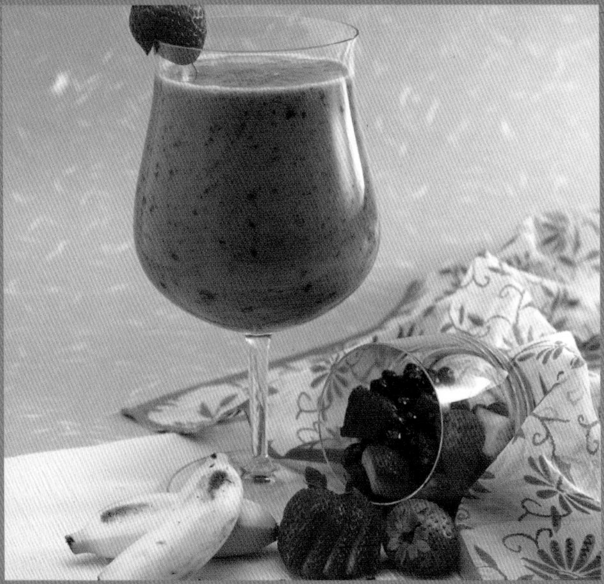

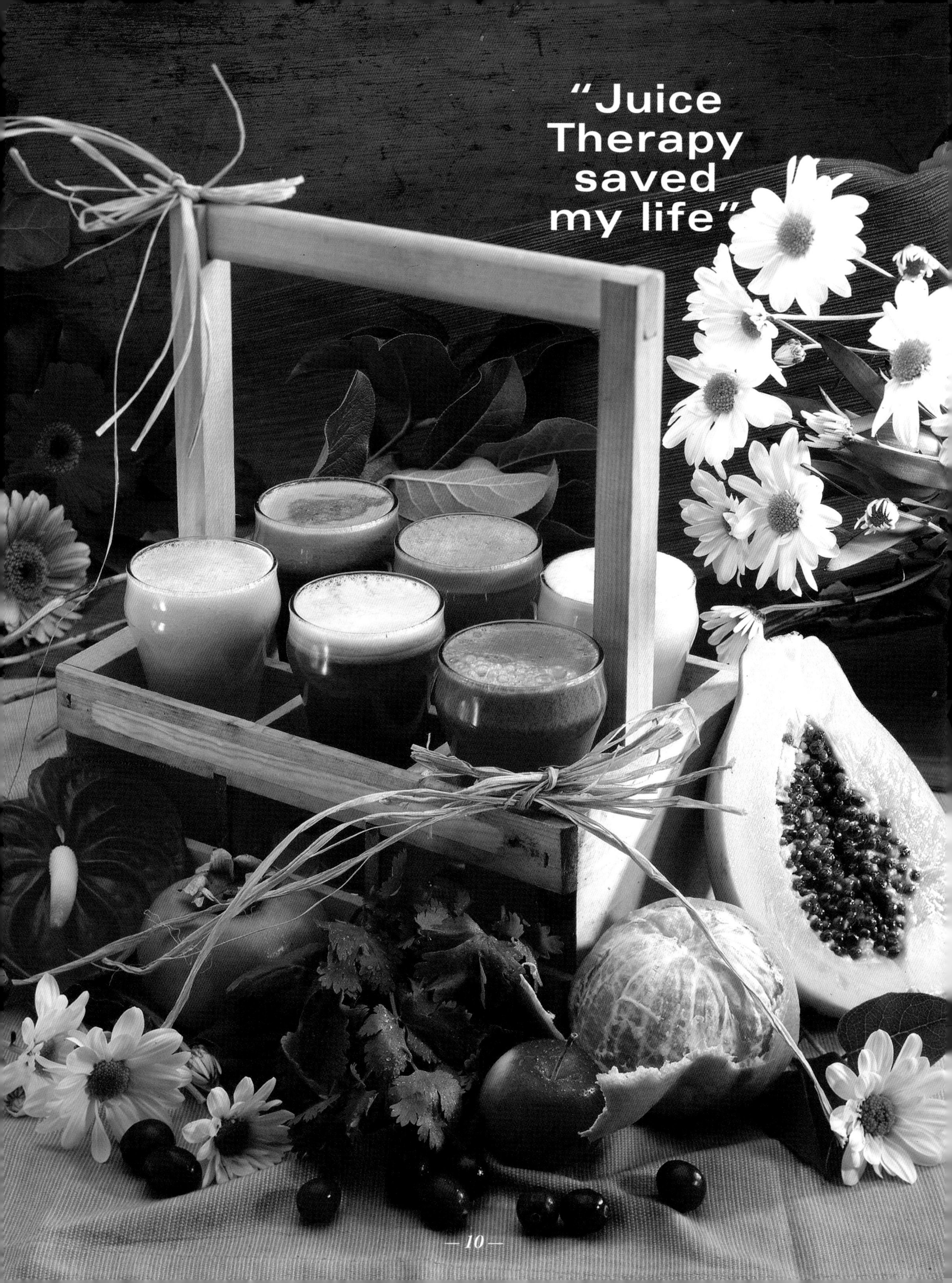
"Juice
Therapy
saved
my life"

Chapter 2

The Power of Juicing

- Jay's life's story: How he Survived Cancer
- Why Juicing is so Important
- Jay's *Quick-Start* 3 Day Juice Fast
- Jay's Top Twelve Juice Therapy Recipes
- Children's Favorite Super Juices
- Jay's Special Digestive Juice Tonics

Healing Juices

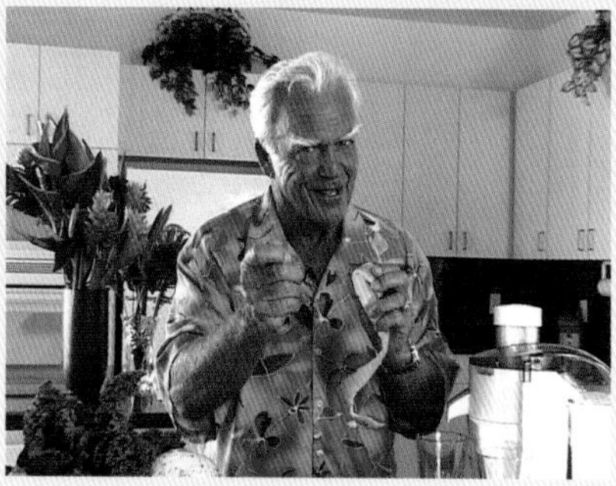

Did you ever wonder why juicing has always been so important to me? In my first book I wrote back in 1992, (#1 on the New York Times Best Seller List) The Power of Juicing, I didn't get a chance to discuss much, other than to share many juicing recipes with you. If you haven't heard my life's story before, you can hear it on my audio tape, titled *My Life's Story: How I Beat the Odds*. However, I will briefly discuss it here. Juicing saved my life.

When I was twenty-five, playing football for the University of Southern California in 1947, I pulled a thigh muscle that threw me out of the game for an entire year. During that time, I became sick with a bladder problem that was later diagnosed as bladder cancer. I was told I had less than a year to live, or if I chose, I could go under the knife to have the tumor cut out and receive cobalt treatments. (Back in the 1940s, chemotherapy and radiation had not yet been thoroughly developed.) Cancer amongst Americans was very low in the 1940's. (Unfortunately, now more than one million Americans get diagnosed per year.)

I Made a Big Move

I opted for another choice. I had heard of a medical doctor named Max Gerson, who was becoming an expert at healing cancer through what most people knew about in Europe; Juice Therapy. I quickly went to visit Dr. Gerson, who at that time ran a busy cancer clinic in New York. He agreed to treat me—but only after scolding me about my eating habits and telling me how drastically I had to change my life in order to get well. I eagerly agreed, and thus began a juicing program that went on for three months, (three weeks of which were grueling.) After all, I was taught by my football coach to eat steaks, cakes, and hamburgers every day. The first three weeks on Dr. Gerson's program were almost unbearable. Yet, surprisingly, after those few weeks my body, mind, and soul soon took on an almost euphoric feeling. I lost weight, my skin started to clear up, I wasn't constipated any longer and I could breathe clearly. Most importantly, I wasn't bleeding in the genital area any longer. I began to have hope for my future. After all I was only 25 years old. Before those three weeks, I had been bleeding every day while urinating.

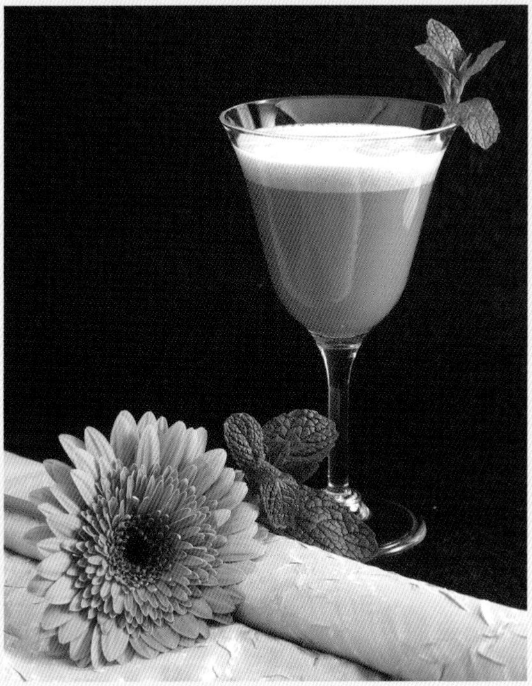

What to Juice – What to Eat?

After three months of Dr. Gerson's treatments, I went home and continued on my own, fasting on juices for another two years. I sipped warm broths in the winter months, and, eventually, I started adding more organic, pure foods to my diet. Even now, I consume mostly raw, unadulterated, organic fruits and vegetables. You could say that I mostly eat fruit and juice my vegetables. Why? It's very simple. Fruits mostly consist of natural mineral water. For example, here are some fruits I recommend to eat or blend:

- Papaya (without skin)
- Mango (without skin)
- Banana (without skin)
- All Berries
- Stone fruits (with skin)
- Kiwis (with or without skin)
- Cantaloupe (without skin)
- Watermelon (without skin)
- Grapes with skins*
- Coconut (without shell-drink the water)
- Pineapples (without skin)

**Only eat grapes with seeds-they have not been hydribidized and have more nutrients.*

Below are the fruits we love to eat too, but we also recommend juicing these fruits.

- Apples with skins
- Pineapples (without the peel)
- Pears (extra firm-if soft, we eat them)
- Oranges (without skin-but peel thinly)
- All melons (with skins only if organic)
- Grapefruits (without peel-but peel thinly)

Apples are not good blended, yet pineapples, pears and oranges blend well, but we prefer to eat these fruits because they have less water content than the others and they are rich with fiber, as our bodies need large amounts of daily in order to function at its optimum.

My Mission Begins

My cancer scare in the 1940s started me on a mission to teach others about the healing power of juice therapy. I gave up my studies at USC, unfortunately only a few credits short of receiving my bachelors of science degree. Obviously I gave up a rich football career and lifestyle for this commitment, and I'm so grateful I did. I have spent the last fifty-seven years traveling across North America extolling the virtues of juicing, and my life is richer than before, blessed with health, vitality, and happiness even now in the year 2005. Even though I lost my precious trademark and ability to teach for ten years, I still consider myself blessed with wonderful, vital health everyday. When you don't have your health, it doesn't matter how rich, happy, or successful you are. Illness has a way of stopping everything in its tracks.

Juicing is a Serious Subject

It's personally heartbreaking to see people purchase juicers and end up using them occasionally for alcoholic drinks or for fun at parties. Juicing is a very serious subject, one that I have spent my entire life dedicated to, and, ultimately, teaching. Linda and I are content knowing many Americans are purchasing more and more juicers, but without knowing what 'Juice Therapy" truly is, we believe it's like having a car without gas. Since 1993, I have not been able to publish books on juicing, due to trademark challenges; otherwise, I would have written many more juicing books. However, now you can be rest assured, before I leave this Earth, Linda and I will share as much as we can, despite publishing challenges.

You Can have Energy like I Do

In step with this fact, I would like you to trust in my ability to teach and guide you in helping you achieve the kind of vital energy I feel everyday. For example, Dr. Gabriel Cousins, my personal medical Doctor emphasizes most carrots are hybridized, and contain more sugar in them than during the years I treated my own cancer. He is the leading medical authority on Living Foods in the world. With that thought in mind, I now only recommend juicing my famous carrot/apple combination with 80% carrots and only 20% apples, unlike my original recipes which recommended 50/50. I also recommend minimizing your fruit juice intake to mornings. Blood sugar issues can be helped, particularly when juicing Brussels Sprouts and string beans together. See Chapter 5 for more information on the Pancreas. According to Dr. Norman Walker in his book, *Raw Vegetable Juicing*, this combination is almost identical to the natural insulin our bodies manufacture. I highly recommend you read this book, since Dr. Walker was one of my mentors. This man practiced what he preached and knew a tremendous amount about the powers of juice therapy. He died disease free at an age of over 100 back in 1984.

It was Dr. Gerson and Dr. Walker who lead me to the powerful path of Juice Therapy and Living Foods. Now that they are gone, I feel it is now my job to teach to you these ageless, health-building truths.

The Real Juicing Advantage

As you are about to discover, fresh, living juice is a veritable powerhouse—rich with vitamins, minerals, living enzymes, and phytochemicals—all of which have an extraordinarily healthful and beneficial effect on your body. If you don't make fresh juices at home and drink them within an hour, you will lose these precious enzymes, vital to building energy and superior digestion. If you cannot do this because of time constraints, I recommend purchasing fresh juices from the grocery store. However, don't be fooled when you go to the grocery store to purchase fresh juices. Read the labels carefully to make sure these juices are not pasteurized and that they are organic. If you live in a large city, purchasing fresh juice from juice bars is a wonderful way to get your fresh juice. When Linda and I travel to Hawaii every summer to give lectures on living foods and juicing, we always stop by my good friend Pablo's juice bar - Lanikai Juice. If you are ever in Kailua, Hawaii, stop by and get juiced up – they've got great juice combinations and wonderfully tasting fresh organic fruits.

The Magic of Juice Therapy

The magic of juicing is that it instantly releases these life-giving nutrients, and here's the clincher—renders them "*body-active*" in about fifteen minutes. Do you know how long it takes to digest a typical American meal, say steak, potatoes and salad? Try more than six and one half hours. And during that process, a lot of the nutrients are lost. The bulk, especially the hard-to-digest sinewy meat (which can actually remain in your system one, two, or even three days or more), can prevent all of the important nutrients from being absorbed. Notwithstanding the putrifaction that takes place while all that food is stuck in your intestines. The key to good health is fast elimination. Fruits digest themselves without needing any enzymes, and this is all done within 20 minutes after consuming. This is why most of us get hungry after eating fruit. If you eat a primarily living foods diet, most of our foods are eliminated with 17 hours of consumption. When the body does not have to work hard to digest, guess what? We have more energy. We feel more alive! We have time to enjoy our lives, instead of crashing at 8pm in front of the television.

Juicing Gives us 100% Absorption Immediately

When you juice, you get almost 100 percent of the food's value concentrated in dense, nutrient-rich, liquid form, pre-digested. Like fruit, fresh juice digests itself, without having to rob enzymes from another part of the body. You see, juicing gives you the highest density of nutrients per calorie. Eating food is simplistic. Juicing goes many steps further, releasing *all* of the food's value, just the way nature intended in the beginning.

New scientific research shows most, perhaps 90 percent, of fruit and vegetable food value lies not in the flesh, but in the peelings and just below the surface. And that, you see, is the real juicing advantage. Juicing is nature's key, unlocking and releasing nutrients that are normally unavailable because of our inability to eat things that are indigestible, like the rind of the watermelon, or the outer skin of a pineapple.

It is precisely because the fiber is left behind that fresh, raw juice is the best source of instant nutrition for your body. What's more, freshly made juices are delicious. In fact, if you've never had "*real*" juice before, you are in for quite a treat. There is absolutely nothing like it. In our opinion, there simply is no superior beverage to be had on Earth.

The Mysteries of Life-giving Plants

Do you know where enzymes, vitamins, and minerals come from? Minerals are formed in the under layers of the earth's crust. Plants literally *drink* them up from the soil. Indeed, it would be another matter entirely if you could grab a handful of rich earth, eat it, and absorb the iron, phosphorus, calcium, zinc, and boron. But we can't. Only plants have the propensity to draw minerals up through their roots and to absorb the sun's energy, through photosynthesis, metamorphosing them into the plants' cellular walls.

Dr. Walker explains further: "*The rays of the sun send billions of atoms into plant life, activating the enzymes, and by this force, they change inorganic*

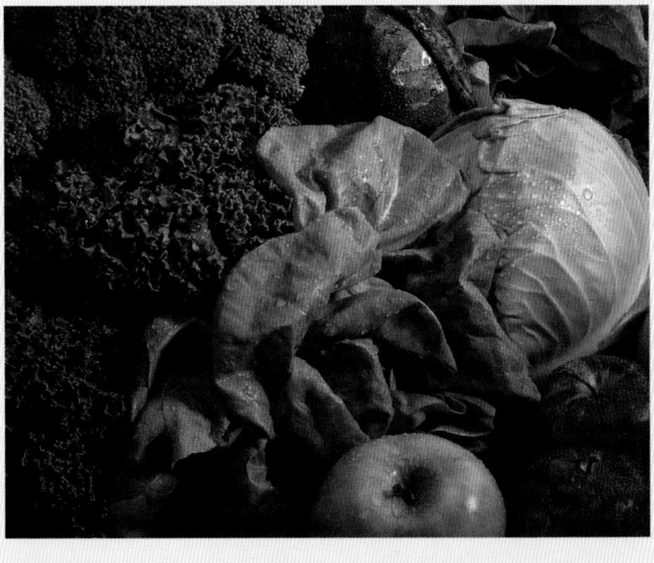

elements into organic or life-containing elements for food." If we cook our foods, this life-force is extinguished.

Likewise, enzymes and vitamins— the spark plugs of life—are manufactured in the cell walls of plant tissue. They are literally bound within the plant, *locked into the living fibers*. So the vital parts of fruits and vegetables— that which contains the greatest concentrated value of nutriments—is the most difficult to reach. Juicing is the key to unlocking and releasing the full spectrum of *live nourishment*: liquid Mother Nature pours forth when you juice live fruits and vegetables. That's why I've said for more than fifty-five years:

> *"It's the juice of the fiber that feeds you!"*

In this age of pervasive pollution from our toxic environment, to chemically treated water supplies, to processed, refined, adulterated foods we eat—juicing is the key to internal body cleansing. Juicing has the power to give you a full body makeover, rebuilding your youth from the inside out.

Getting Started

Now that you know why juicing is so important, I invite you to cleanse your system and fast like I have been doing for many years. The following method is a great way to start. Juice fasting is a very powerful, yet cathartic, experience, and there are some techniques I have learned over the years that may help you during this juice fast that I now present to you in this chapter.

Before you Start your Cleanse

1. Before beginning any juice fasting program, you should consult your health-care practitioner or medical doctor, especially if you are hypoglycemic.
2. If you have a three day holiday coming up, this would be the most opportune time to start.
3. Rest your body, mind and soul during these three days, exercising lightly.
4. Please rid your kitchen of any foods that may dissuade you from your commitment to these three days.
5. Purchase enough water for the 3 day cleanse, which is approximately eight, 10-ounce (250-milliliter) glasses of pure water daily. We drink steam distilled water only. If you can find Trinity Mineral Water, we highly suggest using it. It is the only other water we drink. If you go to trinityspring.com you will find their web site. This is the purest water we have ever found, and we recommend it highly.
6. If you absolutely need to eat something during your fast, peel an orange, slowly eat it, and spit out the pulp after you have masticated it thoroughly in your mouth.
7. Take a natural laxative every day to help move the bowels, since you won't be eating any food. Because bowel/intestinal cleansers can pull moisture from your body more than usual, there is a need to drink more water during your fast.
8. Slow down your work pace. Use these times for relaxation, contemplation and prayer/meditation, reading, walking, yoga, and stretching. You should exercise at least 30 minutes daily, by walking, stretching, or yoga. At the end of the day, Linda finds a relaxing bath at night with lavender oil really helps. I prefer a warm shower, either after waking or before retiring. Before showering or bathing, use a dry body brush to massage your skin for five minutes. This stimulates the largest organ of your body, your skin, helping it to breathe and to stimulate the blood flow to all your pores.

I usually fast once every six months for approximately seven days. Sometimes it's only three or four days, depending on how I am feeling, or the season. We need to listen to our body. Over time, it will not betray us.

My 3 Day Quick-Start Cleanse:

- **Morning: fresh fruit juice (see recipes), diluted 50/50 with pure water**
- **Mid-morning: cup of organic herbal tea such as chamomile, peppermint or ginger.**
- **Lunch: fresh vegetable juice (see recipes)—24 ounces**
- **Mid-afternoon: more vegetable juice or more water.**
- **Dinner: fresh vegetable juice—24 ounces**
- **Evening: cup of herbal tea, preferably chamomile**
- **Drink steam distilled water throughout the day (between two and three liters)**

Important Rules:

1. Please do not use sweeteners of any kind during your fast.
2. When you are drinking tea, make sure it is not too hot.
3. Do not drink any kind of stimulating teas such as green tea or black tea.
4. Ensure all your produce is thoroughly washed and organically grown.
5. Drink approximately eight glasses (two liters) of fresh juice daily in addition to at least five glasses (1.25 liters) of water. We like to add a squeeze of organic lemon to water, making it alkaline.

Following are some of my favorite freshly made juice combinations, depending on the season. Each recipe makes about two cups (500 milliliters).

Fruit Juice Recipe for Fasting

Grapefruit-Ginger-Apple: Peel one medium sized grapefruit, leaving most of the white pulp in tact. Use one-half inch of ginger, not peeled. Use three golden delicious apples (to help counteract the tartness of the grapefruit).

Cranberry-Apple-Pineapple: Use a handful of fresh cranberries, two apples, and one-half pineapple. (Peel the hard skin off before juicing.)

Apple-Blueberry: Place one cup (250 grams) fresh blueberries, alternating with four golden delicious apples (so the blueberries do not fly up and hit the ceiling!).

Remember: When you are choosing to use fruit juices during this fast, it is sometimes important to dilute these juices 50/50 with pure water (steam distilled), or Trinity water. Sometimes fruit juices can be very cleansing, causing a fast detoxifying reaction. Also, if you have blood sugar issues, we suggest using fruit juices only diluted with water, and only once per day. When you dilute your juices with water, it can ease the detoxifying process. Also, try to remember to only purchase organic fruits and vegetables. We purchase some of our organic food online through www.boxedgreens.com.

Fresh Vegetable Juice Combination for Fasting

When we talk about vegetable juices, I usually mean any of the following combinations of vegetables, consisting of approximately 75 percent carrot, and the rest, any dark greens you wish to use such as broccoli, bok choy, kale, spinach, endive, parsley, or wheat grass. As a rule of thumb, use 70 percent carrot, 20 percent greens, and l0 percent apple. When you become a "vegetable juice" expert, or have blood sugar issues, omit the apple and replace it with l0 percent more greens. Within a while you can get up to 60 percent carrot and 40 percent greens. When you are juicing with vegetables, remember to start with firmer vegetables such as carrots. It allows the more tender greens and softer vegetables to flow through faster and more efficiently.

Carrot-Spinach-Apple-Beet: Use eight carrots, a small handful of spinach, three apples, and one-quarter of a beet without greens. Because beets are so incredibly potent, please be careful when you use them. Another rule, never use more than 30% percent beets in any combination of juices, whether it be strictly with apples or vegetables. You may use the beet greens only if the beets are organic, and when you have at least thirty days of vegetable and beet juicing behind you. Beet greens are very cleansing, so we want to make sure you understand to take it a bit slowly. Another tip on juicing with beets: If your urine and stools appear red, please don't be concerned. This always seems to alarm people! It's just the red pigment from the beets coming through your body. If you get gaseous, don't worry; it's just your liver cleaning out toxins. If it persists, cut the dose of the beets in half, and start to add more within time, or you may dilute your juices, which greatly helps beginners. Another tip is to only juice the beets and not the greens. Beet greens have a very strong detoxifying effect on your liver and gall bladder. Sometimes diluting the juices with 50% pure, steam distilled water is a great help.

Carrot-Parsley-Spinach-Celery-Apple:

Use about eight carrots, a handful of parsley, a handful of spinach, two apples, and two stalks of celery. Alternate carrots with the greens, because they juice better this way. The carrots flush out the greens that get stuck inside the bowl of the juicer. You may use the apples to do the same job. This is true for all juicers, even if they are the Champion, Acme, Omega, Moulinex, Juiceman or any other juicer.

You may want to play with these different kinds of juice combinations so you can ultimately find the right one for you. If you just remember the basic rules mentioned above, you will learn to be an expert right away - 60-70 percent carrot, and the rest greens with a small apple. Below, you will find Our Digestive Juice Aids which will also be wonderful to add to your juice fasting repertoire!

If you become weak during your juice fast, simply rest and drink plenty of pure water. In the beginning, you may experience the following:

1. Headache
2. Nausea
3. Disorientation or dizziness
4. Diarrhea
5. Weakness and/or achy feeling
6. Pimples or boils
7. Excessive mucus or runny nose
8. Irritability, anger, frustration

These symptoms are the result of beginning stages of detoxification, and this explains the need for water throughout the day, despite your juicing regime. You may even want to dilute your juices to help ease the process, which we recommend. After the second or third day, you will start to feel great. If you don't, please consult your doctor or your health practitioner.

Congratulations

You have finished your juice fast. Congratulate yourself and those who have supported and loved you through it. Many people are addicted to foods, and you have accomplished something few can actually do. Break your fast with light foods such as fruits and salads without a lot of dressing for the next few days. Try to understand that your body has just cleansed itself of a lot of built-up toxin. (See pages 20-21) for Digestive Juicing recipes.

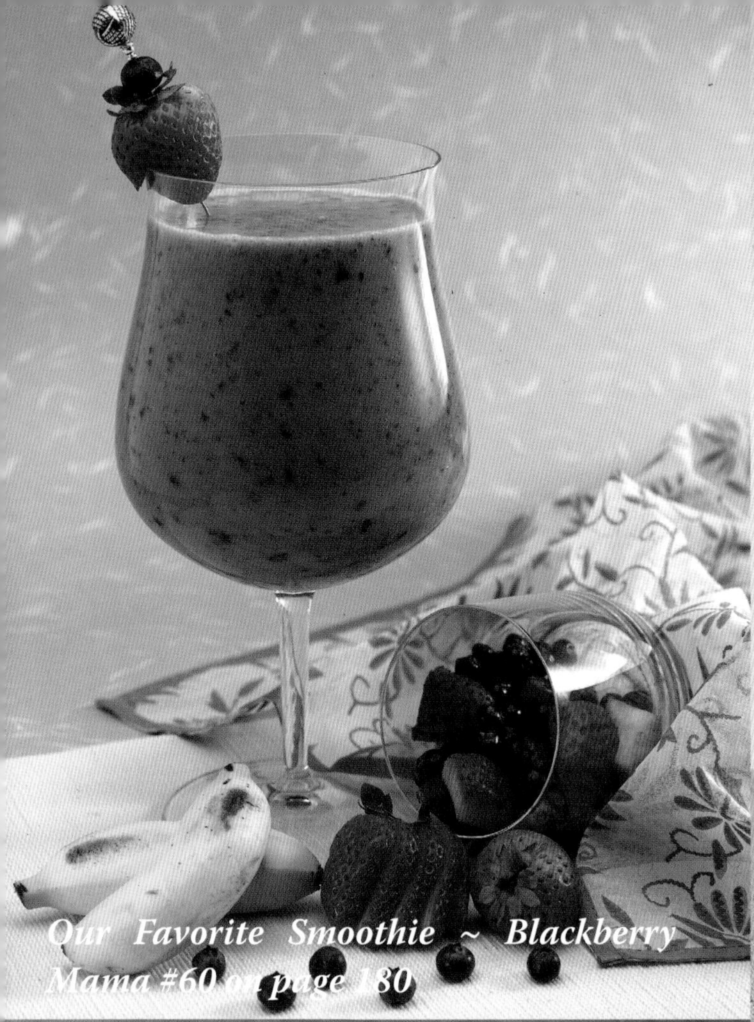

Our Favorite Smoothie ~ Blackberry Mama #60 on page 180

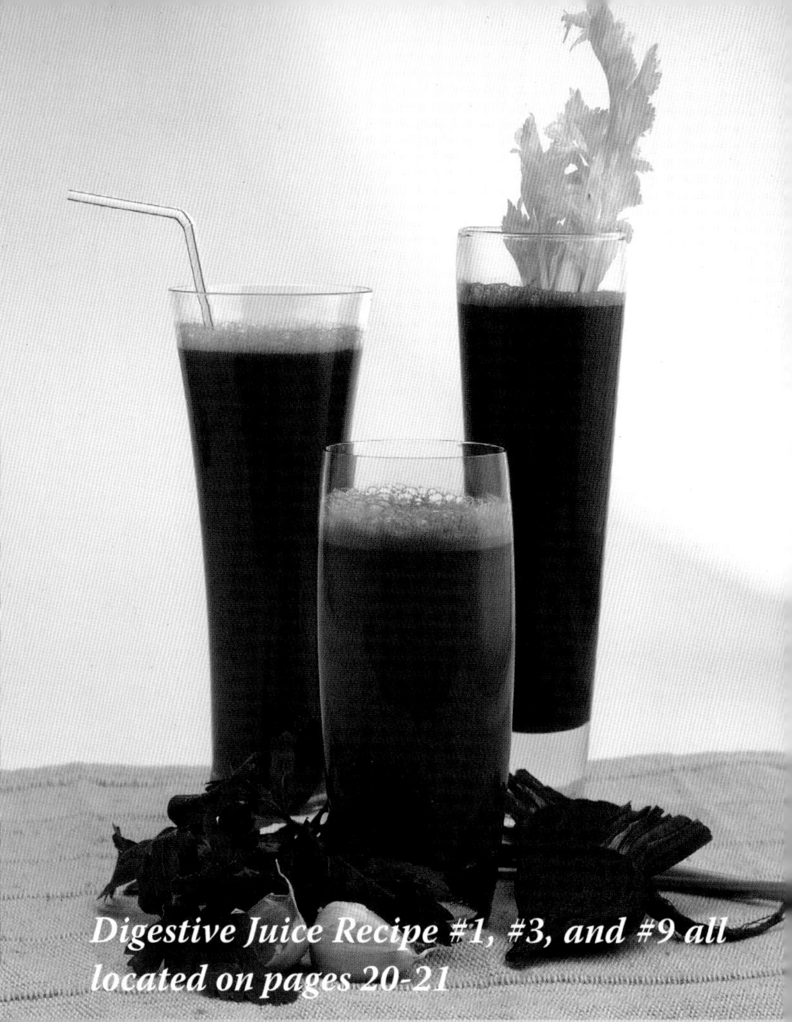

Digestive Juice Recipe #1, #3, and #9 all located on pages 20-21

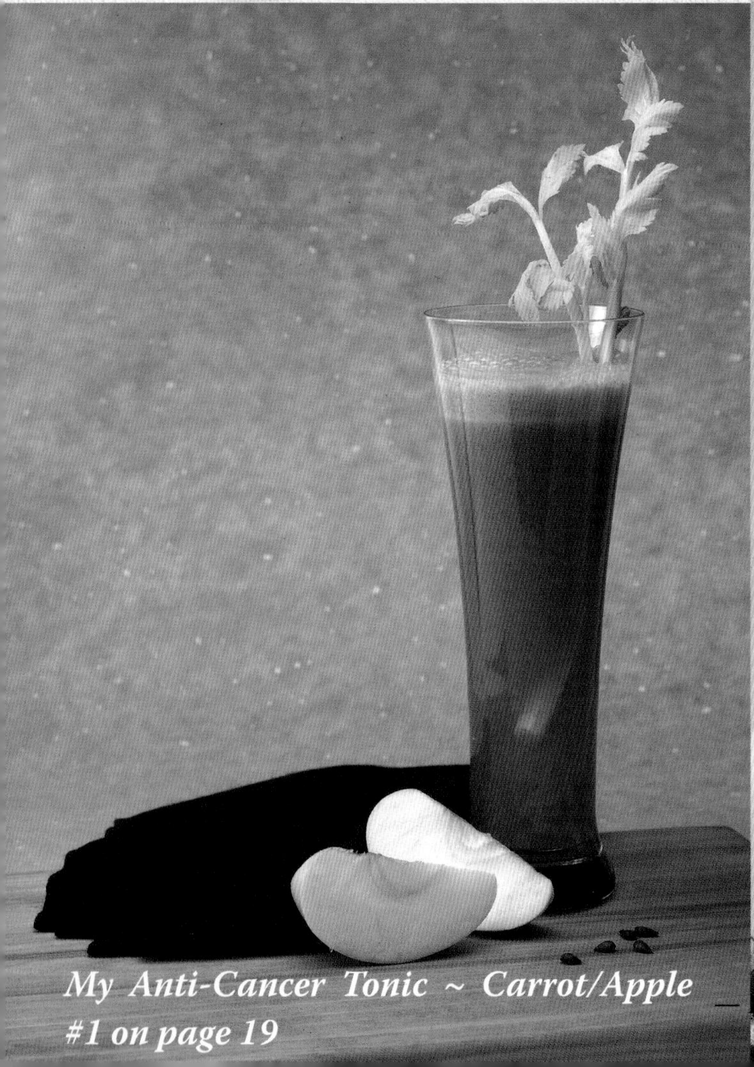

My Anti-Cancer Tonic ~ Carrot/Apple #1 on page 19

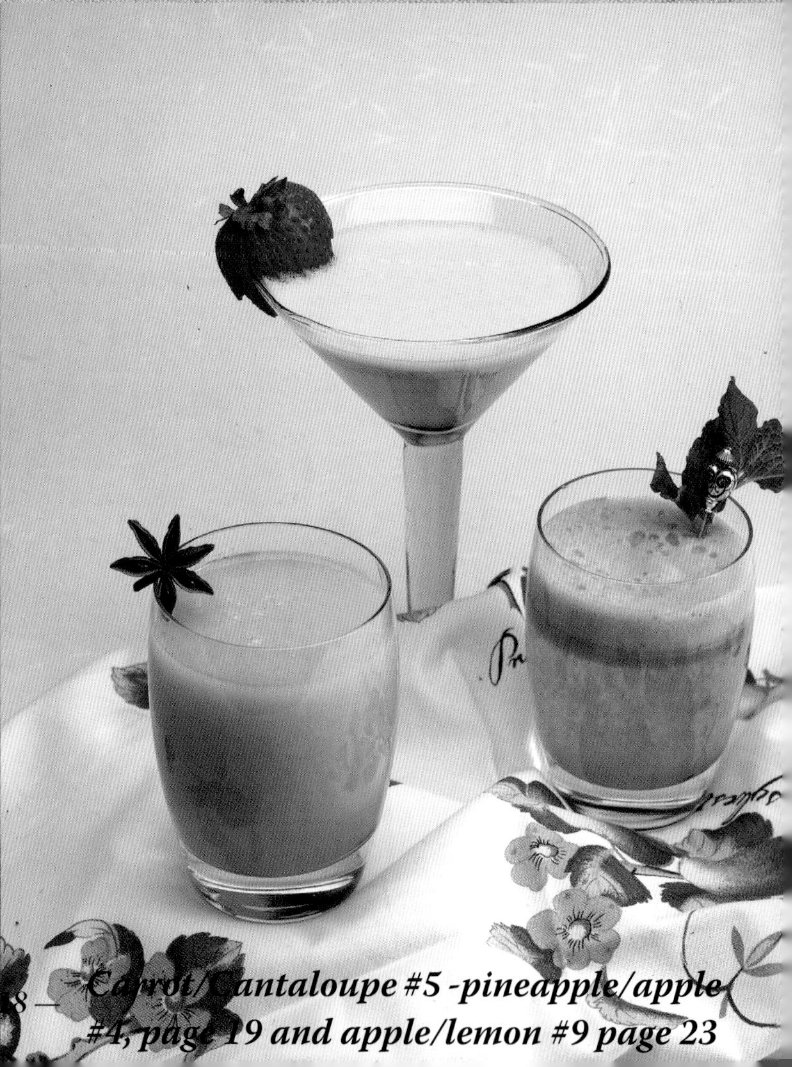

Carrot/Cantaloupe #5 -pineapple/apple #4, page 19 and apple/lemon #9 page 23

It is important to treat your body well. By accomplishing this feat, you now have the ability to help heal your body by juice fasting at will. Whenever you need to restore your vital energy lost through poor food choices and stressful living, you can turn to the healing power of juice fasting. When you are not fasting and want to incorporate juicing into your daily regime, these are some of my favorite recipes. I've used these recipes for the last fifty-seven years.

Here are My Top 12 Vital Juice Combinations.

	Juice Combinations	Ingredients	Remedy
1	Carrot/Apple	Six carrots, two Golden Delicious apples.	Dr. Gerson's anti-cancer drink.
2	Apple/Beet	Four red delicious apples, one-half beet with beet greens.	King of the liver cleansers.
3	Carrot/Parsley/Spinach/Celery	Eight medium carrots, a handful of parsley and spinach, and three ribs of celery,	Fantastic digestion tonic.
4	Pineapple/Apple	One-half pineapple, three Golden Delicious apples.	Wonderful for relieving arthritis.
5	Carrot/Cantaloupe (Organic a must)	Eight medium carrots, half cantaloupe with skin. (If not organic, peel the skin.)	Extremely high in antioxidants; wonderful for the skin.
6	Apple/Pear	Five Golden Delicious apples, two pears,	Great to relieve constipation; good drink before bedtime.
7	Carrot/Spinach	Eight medium carrots, handful of spinach	King of healing irritable bowels and digestive troubles.
8	Apple/Celery	Five Golden Delicious apples, three ribs of celery.	Wonderful for relaxation and for after workouts.
9	Watermelon juice with the skin (Organic a must.)	Cut watermelon strips in long, one-inch widths and juice. (If not organic, peel the skin.)	Great for kidney function and good for dehydration.
10	Carrot/Celery/Cabbage	Eight medium carrots, three ribs of celery, one-fourth green cabbage.	The ultimate juice combination for relieving and healing all stomach ulcers
11	Carrot/Endive/Kale/Cucumber	8 medium carrots, one large handful of Endive and Kale, and one large, peeled cucumber.	wonderful for digestion and especially for eye problems. Good for kidneys also
12	Cabbage/Cucumber/Carrot	12 medium sized carrots, 1/4 green cabbage and one large, peeled Cucumber	great for stomach problems, but is also good for cleansing our kidneys.

Please remember to wash and scrub your vegetables at all times before you juice, even if they are organic. Fungus and/or e.coli can grow on cantaloupe and pineapples. Remove all pesticides with a special pesticide remover if not organic!

Our Digestive Juice Aids

	Juice Combinations	Remedy	Ingredients	Preparation Tips
1	Heavy Green Digestive	This juice combination makes an excellent accompaniment to Chinese entrees.	8 medium carrots 3 large leaves Chinese cabbage (Bok Choy) 6 medium broccoli flowerets Handful of spinach	Trim and cut ends of carrots for juicing. Bunch up cabbage leaves and spinach leaves tightly. In the juicer push spinach alternately with carrots. Make sure that the last food pushed through is a carrot, to ensure all spinach juice is extracted.
2	Meal Sipper Digestive	This is one of our favorite juice combinations for aiding digestion	6-8 medium carrots Handful of spinach leaves	Trim and cut ends of carrots. Bunch up spinach leaves tightly. In a juicer
3	**Salad Tonic Digestive**	If you are eating a more predominately cooked meal we suggest you use this recipe. It substitutes for a salad and it's got great digestive aid properties.	8 medium carrots 3 beet top leaves l clove garlic l/2 beet sliced One large tomato 2 stalks celery 3 medium broccoli flowerets 2 radishes	Trim and cut ends of carrots and tightly bunch up beet top leaves. In a juicer place the garlic first followed by the beet leaves. Follow up with carrots.Juice the remaining ingredients.
4	Basic Digestive Tonic	This is also good for stomach ailments, but also wonderful as a diuretic for swelling in our bodies due to excess salt intake.	8 medium carrots l handful of spinach 2 stalks celery	Trim and cut ends of carrots, and tightly bunch up spinach. In a juicer, push spinach through alternately with carrots. Juice celery and finish juicing remaining carrots, if any.
5	Blood Building Digestive	Wonderful for building strong iron in our bloodstreams. It is also a blood cleanser and stomach reliever.	8 medium carrots Handful kale Handful spinach 1 apple, quartered	Trim and cut ends of carrots. Tightly bunch up kale and spinach. In a juicer, push kale and spinach through, alternately with carrots; juice apples, and finish juicing with any remaining carrots.
6	Digestive Calming Tonic	We use this juice combination at night, before we retire, if we are stressed out. This is also very good as a digestive aid with any cooked meal.	8 carrots Handful spinach 2 stalks celery Handful parsley	Trim and cut ends of carrots. Tightly bunch up spinach and parsley. In a juicer, push spinach and parsley through alternately with carrots. Then alternate juicing the celery, apples, and carrots.

	Juice Combinations	Remedy	Ingredients	Preparation Tips
7	Digestive Companion	Spinach is the king of remedies for stomach ailments. It alleviates all problems with either diarrhea or constipation.	8 medium carrots Handful spinach 1 apple	Trim and cut ends of carrots. Tightly bunch up spinach. In a juicer, push spinach alternately through with carrots and proceed with apple.
8	Green Power Tummy Remedy	Wonderful for relieving stomach aches due to overeating. Ginger addition adds to more power to better digestion.	8 medium carrots Handful spinach Handful parsley 2 stalks celery 1-inch thick fresh ginger root	Trim and cut ends of carrots. Tightly bunch up spinach and parsley. In a juicer, push spinach and parsley alternately through with carrots, ginger, and celery.
9	Green Tummy Machine	King of the digestion remedies. Cabbage combined with the spinach is great for relieving indigestion and heartburn	8 medium carrots Handful kale Handful spinach Handful green cabbage 1 apple	Trim and cut ends of carrots. Tightly bunch up kale and spinach. In a juicer, alternately push kale and spinach with the carrots. Juice the apples, cabbage, and finish with any remaining carrots
10	Popeye's Digestive Special Serves 1	Good iron tonic and liver cleanser. Fantastic for helping digest cooked meals.	8 medium carrots Handful fresh spinach 1/4 medium sized beet with beet greens	Trim and cut ends of carrots. Tightly bunch up spinach. In a juicer, push spinach alternately with half the carrots. Finish with beets and their greens and the remaining carrots.
11	Power Up Digestive	A sweet drink, and wonderful for children who do not like to eat cooked veggies. this is a wonderful remedy for relieving any swelling in the hands or feet, and good for digestion too.	8 medium carrots Handful fresh spinach 1 cucumber, peeled 1 apple	Trim and cut ends of carrots. Tightly bunch up spinach. In a juicer, push spinach alternately through with carrots, then juice cucumber and apple. Finish with remaining carrots, if any.
12	Three 'Cs' Digestive	This is one of Jay's favorite juice combinations. It's extremely excellent for stomach ulcers. Very alkaline, this particular combination is used in hospitals throughout the world to cure digestive problems and ulcers.	8 medium carrots 2 stalks celery 1/4 green cabbage	Trim ends of carrots. In a juicer, alternate carrots, celery, and cabbage. Finish with remaining carrots, if any.

Note about Greens

Because greens have highly concentrated nutrients, green juices (derived from parsley, spinach, and other green vegetables) should always be diluted before drinking. Green juices are a high source of chlorophyll, which metabolizes oxygen in the bloodstream, purifying it and at the same time cleansing the kidneys, liver, and urinary tract. Green juices also stimulate the peristaltic wave in the intestines and move the bowels. Green juices are potent. When you juice green vegetables, make sure only about a quarter of the glass contains green juice.

Incidentally, drinking green juice straight will not cause lasting damage, but it may result in light-headedness and abnormal bowel movements for a day or two. Just as a note; if you have trouble with carrots or cannot find them in your area, we suggest you substitute cucumbers for carrots, but instead of using, as an example, 8 carrots in a recipe, cut it in half and only use four cucumbers instead. In some countries around the world, carrots are difficult to find, and also people who are very sensitive to sugar tend to have much better success using cucumbers as a replacement

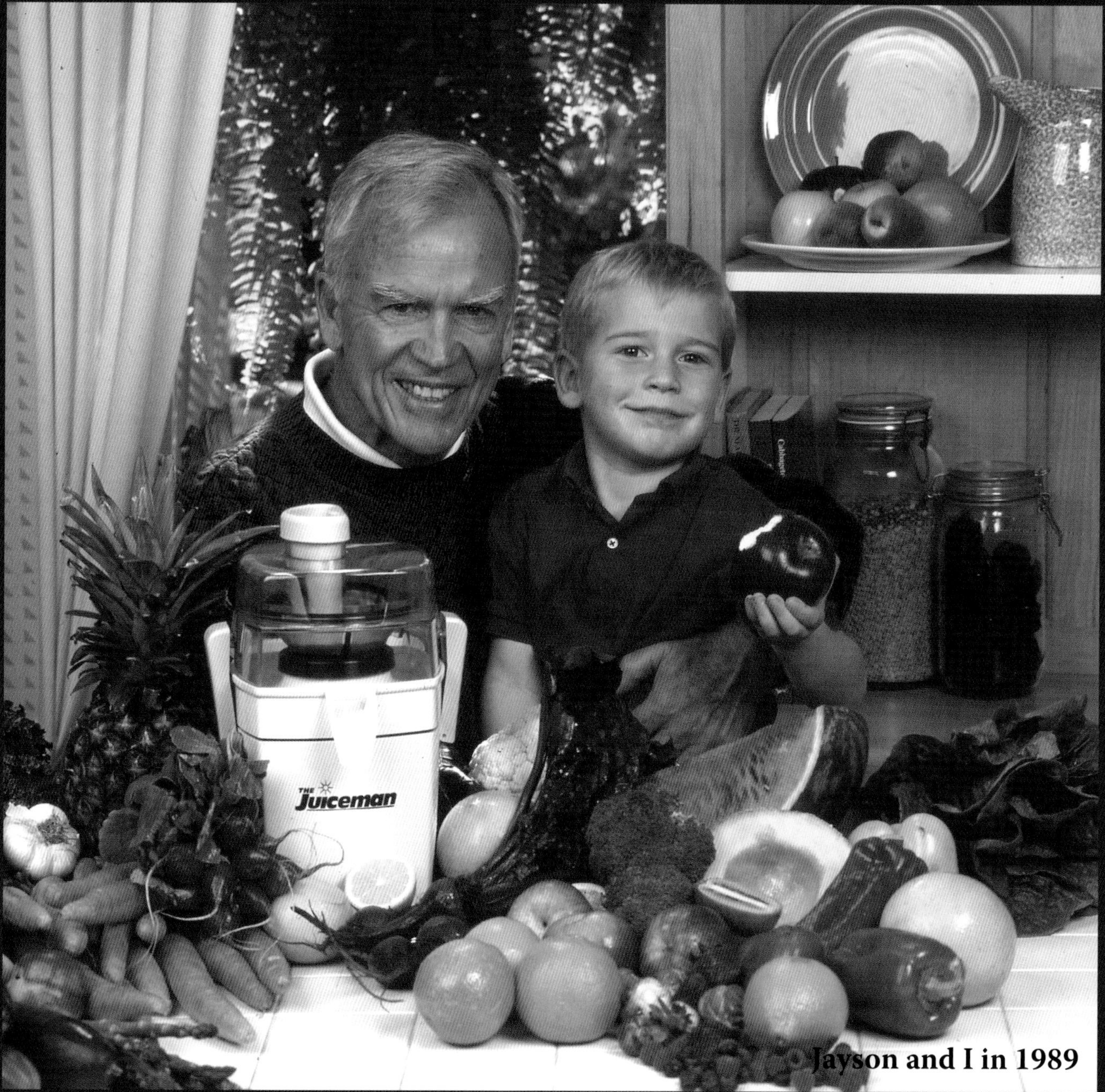

Jayson and I in 1989

Juices For Kids!

Children usually don't like vegetables, but juicing them is a fast and effective way to insure they get all the phytochemicals, vitamins and minerals, enzymes and iron needed in their daily diets. The best way to mask vegetable tastes is to use apples. Also, if they balk at the color, try putting a colored cup or glass in the front of the juicer spout, so the colors are masked.

Children's Top 10 Super Juice Recipes

	Juice Name	*Ingredients*	*Recipe*	*Juice for ages*
1.	Sweet Popeye	Apple/Spinach	4 golden delicious apples to 1/2 cup baby spinach	(Ages 3-19)
2.	Sunshine Delight	Carrot/Apple	8 carrots to 2 golden delicious apples	(ages 2-19)
3.	Bedtime Buddy	Apple/Pear	4 apples (fuji or red delicious) to one firm Pear	(ages 2-19)
4.	Relaxing Charlie	Celery/Apple	3 ribs celery to 2 apples	(ages 2 to 19)
5.	Blue Sky Dreams	Lemon/Grape	3 apples (Pippin) to 1/2 lemon with rind to 1/2 cup dark grapes (Riber grapes or dark red grapes with seeds)	(ages 2-19)
6.	Sweet Bubbles	Orange/Pineapple	2 peeled Oranges to 1/4 Pineapple (without rind, unless organic)	(ages 1.5-19)
7.	Purple Playmate	Blueberry/Orange	1/2 cup fresh Blueberries to 3 peeled Oranges	(ages 1.5 to 19)
8.	Pinky Surprise	Watermelon	one inch sliced watermelon with rind, unless it's not organic. If it's not organic, then peel the red meat from the watermelon and discard rind.	(ages 2-19)
9.	Lemonade Pal	Apple/Lemon	(Jay's Lemonade) 4 Golden Delicious Apples to 1/2 Lemon with rind, unless not organic.	(ages 1.5 to 19)
10.	Red Parrot	Apple/Beet	4 Golden Delicious Apples to 1/4 Beet without the greens	(ages 5-19)

"When You're Gr
You're Clean In

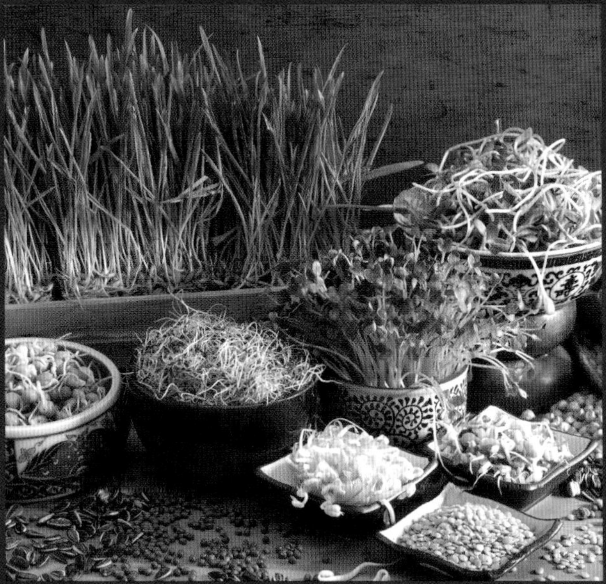

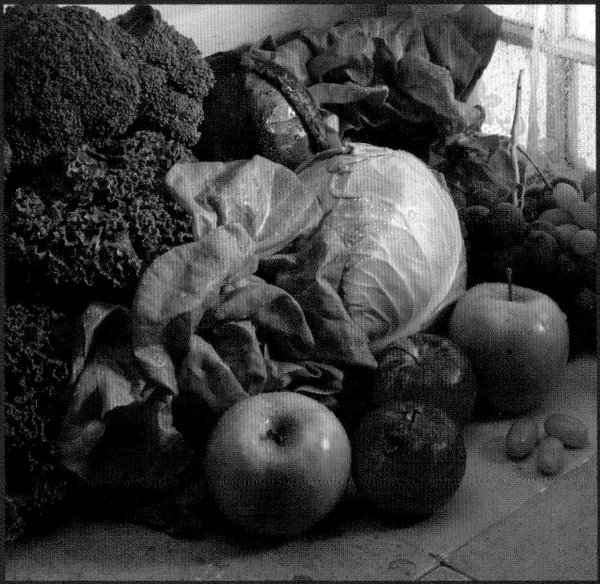

een Inside...
side" *Jay Kordich*

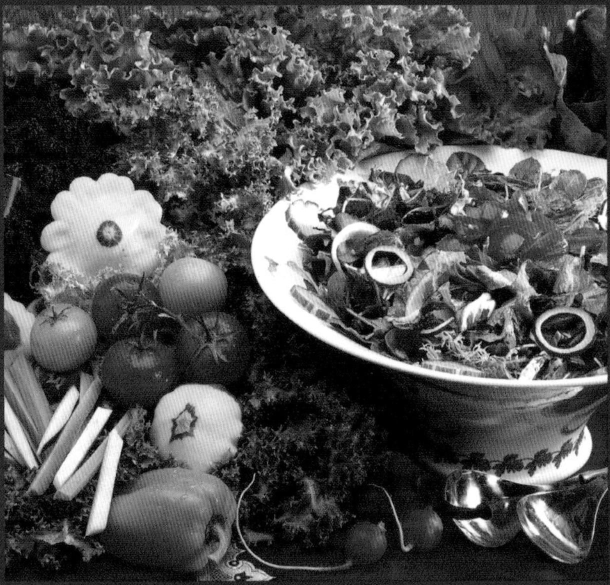

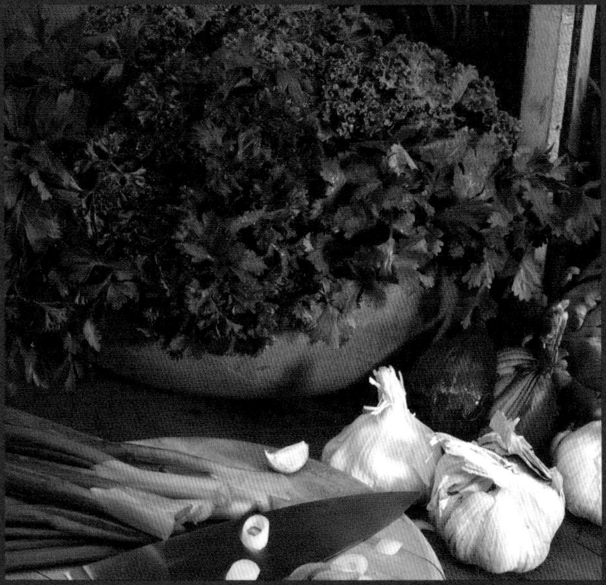

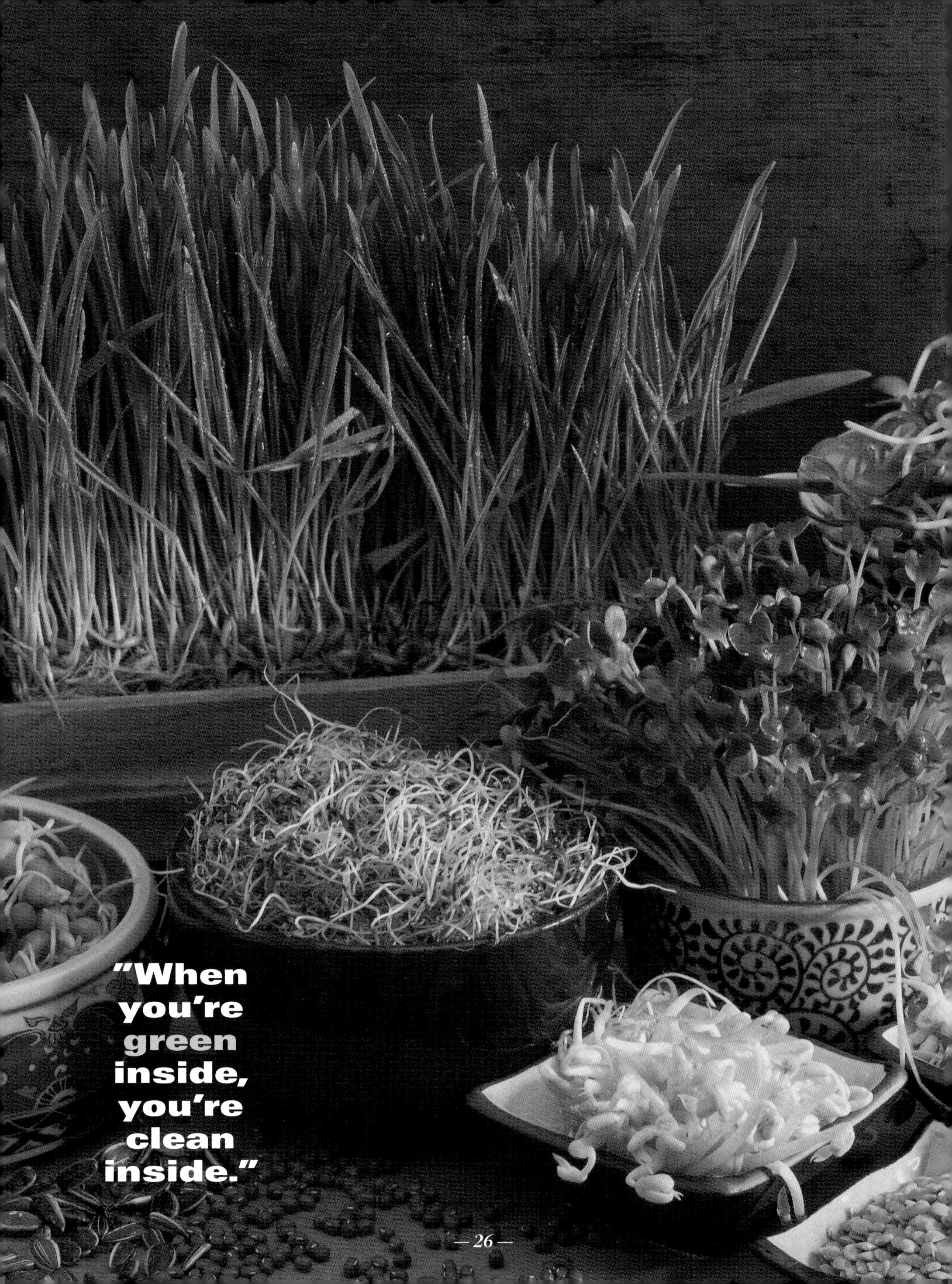

"When you're green inside, you're clean inside."

Color me Green

Take the test— how *GREEN* are you?
How to get 'Un-addicted' from Destructive food habits in Ten Days
How to Color yourself Green - Daily
Detoxification and the Power of Greens
How to De-stress your Life Easily

What is Life-force?

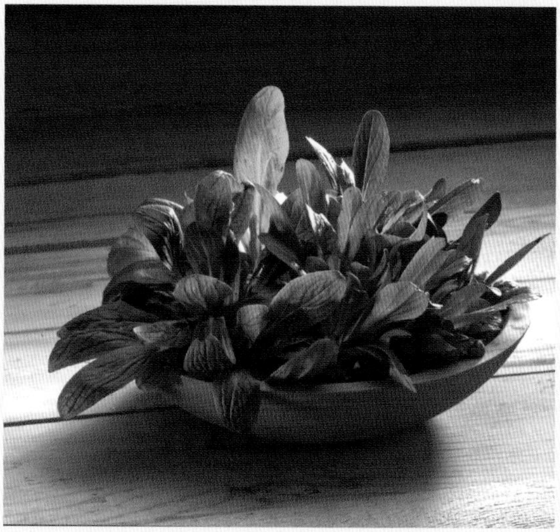

Most of my entire adult life, I have been saying, "All life on planet Earth emanates from the green of the plant." What do I mean by this? First, I would like to say, we underestimate the power of the sun and the power of plant life because quite frankly most of us do not understand the relation between the two. Plants are the **real** factories of life. Through photosynthesis, plants, with their roots deeply planted into the ground, draw inorganic elements and minerals from the soil, beautifully and naturally converting them into what I like to call the Life-Force. This is utilized perfectly by humans, including animals who consume them. Our great mother Earth sustains all human life and nurtures us, including our lakes, rivers, streams, oceans, and plant life. Plants, with their roots embedded deeply into the ground, be it the tree trunk or the blade of a single strand of grass, do what no other animal or human can do, and that is to bathe our cells with highly oxygenated and highly powerful green juices, which by the way is almost identical to the human blood in its structure. Green juices or foods derived from plant-life give us a tremendous advantage by supplying us with wonderful amounts of oxygen, chlorophyll, alkalinity, super-immunity, and high water content capabilities that keeps our cells hydrated and alive. The higher the water content in our foods, the less constipated, the less lethargic we feel, and the purer our systems become. Isn't it marvelous?

Plant-Power equals Vital Energy

Plants are crucial to our vital energy and sustenance for our existence, yet we rarely eat them. This is why it's so important that you understand why I consume a variety of greens daily, either through juicing combinations or eating them. You will be amazed when you start adding greens into your daily diet. It is the key to sustaining vital energy, endurance, and longevity. Green plants, and plants in general, are the heartbeat of life itself.

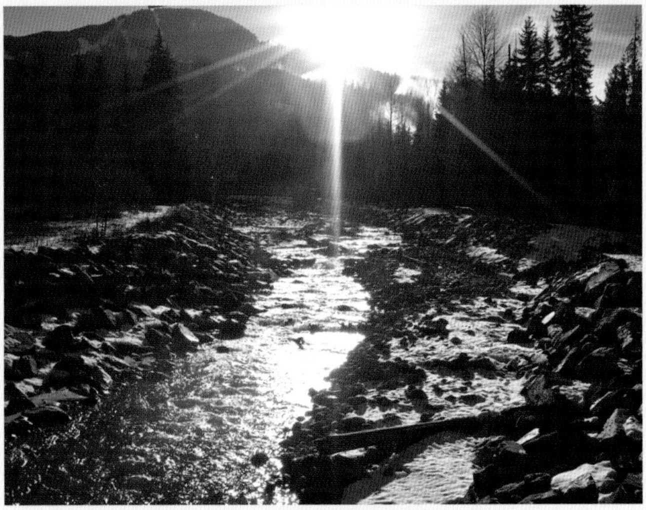

Plants are The Power houses for Humans

Let me explain further: Solar energy and the green of the plant create oxygen on planet Earth for us and all animals to live by. Plants, with their roots dug deep into the ground, draw the inorganic mineral compounds into organic life so we may utilize them as humans. Plants are the factories of life. Erase all plants from the Earth, and we all perish. All food chains begin with plant life. It is in plant life, and the microbes from plants, that nature has brought together all the raw materials required to build, nourish, and sustain life.

How does a cow grow and thrive on a diet of raw grasses? How does a brown bear evolve into such an awe-inspiring magnificent being when the overwhelming majority of its sustenance is raw plant food? The reason is simply this: Plants are live, vital foods vibrating with 'living' enzymes infused with solar energy. This is how we sustain and create energy for the human body. This is why I feel energetic every day, because I have built up a strong immune system abundant with natural vital energy. Even oceans that grow algae and seaweeds, contain huge amounts of powerful super food nutrients. Lit up and infused by the sun's powerful rays, the sun penetrates through the ocean's surface, deep into the depths of the ocean, giving life to the seaweeds. Without the sun, we all perish within a very short span of time.

Our Magnificent Sun

The miracles and magnificence of our sun sometimes goes beyond human understanding, but when you start to consume green foods and super foods via plant life, you will not just be overwhelmed by the immediate infusion of natural energy, you will actually begin to have an innate understanding and natural reverence for this exceptional gift given to us every single day of our lives, as we live on this beautiful blue-green planet of ours.

Plants, and all life on Earth for that matter, require the sun's energy to thrive. Plants derive their energy from the sun during what we've already discussed - photosynthesis. It is in the green of the plant that chlorophyll performs this astounding process, transforming electromagnetic energy (light) into chemical energy, or food. This chemical energy—what fruits and veggies are made of—consists of protein, carbohydrates, essential fatty acids, vitamins, minerals, live enzymes, antioxidants, and phytochemicals, as well as purified plant waters, the most nutritious liquid on Earth.

Liquid Greens are the Key to Life-force

Eating live plants and consuming their juices imbues our bodies with the awesome power of the sun's energy. The late Dr. Amax Bircher-Benner of Europe's world renowned Bircher-Benner clinic was one of the first to advance this truth: *"Absorption and organization of sunlight, the essence of life, takes place almost exclusively within the plants. The organs of the plant are therefore a biological accumulation of light. They are the basis of what we call food, from whence the animal and human body derive their sustenance and energy. Nutritional energy may thus be termed organized sunlight energy. Hence, sunlight is the driving force of the cells of our body."*

Given that our bodies require the sun's energy, and seeing as how plants are the most available form of that energy, doesn't it follow that the most supreme nutrition for the human organism is live plants? Just like animals, humans have a persistent and perpetual need for the vital nutrients that nature has provided in living plant cells. For the human body to function at optimal efficiency and achieve excellent health, it must be supplied with the basic chemicals of life. Our bodies cannot manufacture many of the nutrients we need. We can supply them only in one way: through our diets. When we are under stress of any kind, our bodies burn up the B-complex vitamins, leaving us susceptible to exhausting our delicate nervous system, bringing on many ugly symptoms of emotional instabilities, dysfunctions of the eyes, heart, kidney and liver imbalances. Greens are rich in B Vitamins, including our supergreen smoothie shown here. We add superfoods such as Bee Pollen, Spirulina and Enzymes to our superfood smoothies to ensure we get all the vital nutrients into our bodies daily.

Why Cooking Destroys

In fresh fruits and vegetables, Nature has organized and made available all the raw materials necessary for human life. They are concentrated in all plant bodies in the form of living cells. But as soon as foods are cooked, boiled, or baked or processed, pasteurized and bottled as commercial juice—they are stripped of a vital portion of their nutritive value. Cooking and refining have rendered them inferior forms of nutrition. It is the life-force contained in living plant cells and their rich endowment of nutrients, that sustains, nourishes, and regenerates all the tissues and organs of the human body. In order to be fully utilized as nourishment, those cells must be alive and vital, not cooked and altered.

"Death cannot feed life." This is my life's mission statement: Live Foods Build Live Bodies. Dead foods don't build at all.

Disease Free Living Belongs to ALL

So my dear friends, vital energy and true soul-rewarding experiences are ours for the taking by just acting on and understanding these universal principles. All we have to do is to consume these vital, energetic, viable, and usable plants. Respect the fact that, indeed, the sun and plant life are ours for the taking and the ingesting. As Linda says, your life will change forever. It doesn't have to change overnight. For a few it does, but for most of us, going green takes at least one year to fully integrate.

We're Living a Backwards Life

It is in plant life, and plant life only, that nature has brought together all the raw materials required to build, nourish, and sustain life, including humans. However, if we were to look at reality today regarding our diets here in America, I will tell you, based on recent studies, Americans consume on an average over eight hundred pounds of animal products per year, and most of that is flesh foods. Yet we ignorantly only consume fifteen pounds or more of greens per year. Granted, greens are lighter in weight than animal products, but eight hundred pounds versus fifteen pounds is absurd, yet the truth must be said. It's only through truth can we change, even if the truth hurts or humiliates us.

It's no wonder we are exhausted by the time we reach forty, sick by the time we are fifty, and physically degenerated by the time we are sixty. Most of us have given up and only have small amounts of vital energy left by the time we reach seventy or, luckily, eighty; but some of us don't even reach seventy! It's my belief we are still in middle age by the time we reach sixty, meaning that, we shouldn't really even think of slowing down until we reach seventy-five or eighty. Here I am starting an entirely new business in my mid eighties. The only reason I can do this with Linda is because I have utilized these powerful plants to help feed my body's hundred trillion cells, giving me daily vitality.

When we stay close to nature by consuming the raw foods we were meant to eat such as fruits, berries, nuts, grains, seeds, legumes, vegetables and herbs; we then will have the powers of energy and vitality to sustain us well into our nineties and then some.

My Parents lived a Beautiful Life

My father died at the age of one hundred and three, and my beloved mother passed away at the age of ninety-seven back in 1997. Granted they were not total vegetarians but they lived by the seasons and their yearly garden, ate a tremendous amount of green foods, fresh garlic everyday and lived a very simple, relaxed life. They didn't die of cancer, heart disease, strokes or diabetes like most Americans do. The day my father died was when he ate a large meal with my sisters in San Pedro and came down with a small stomach ache that increased by the time he got home. Within twenty-four hours, he was dead. This is a man who was healthy his entire life, and then one day he just died. What a wonderful way to go. Let's face it, we all have to die, but to die at this age, fully conscious and healthy at the age of 103, that's a very rare event in America now. Most of us are operating at 35% by the time we reach 70, and by the time we reach our 80's we are either bedridden or need to live in an assisted

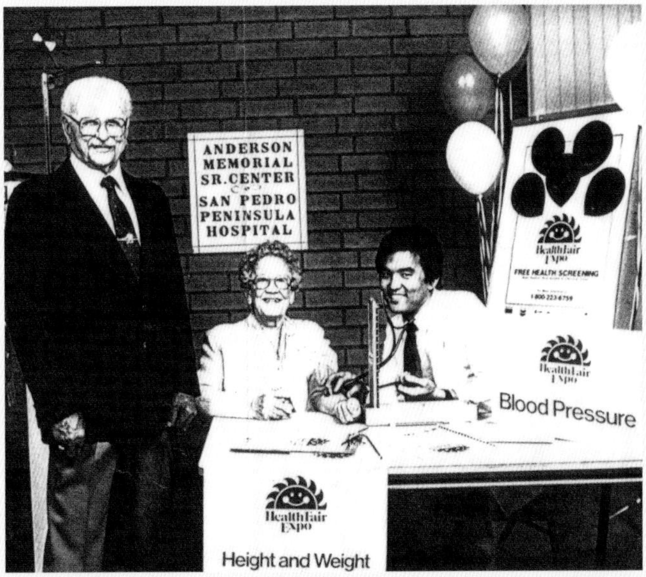

Newspaper article about My Dad at 100 and Mom at 95

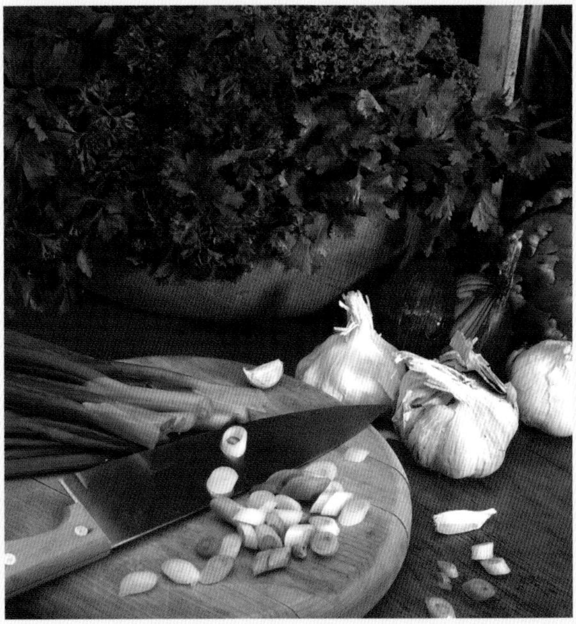

are either bedridden or need to live in an assisted hospital. I *know* we don't have to live this way!

If we simplified our lives, changed our eating habits, ate more greens and tried to live a pure and virtuous life, indeed our lives would change and we will be blessed with a healthy, vital life we are *all* worthy of.

Don't you think its' time for a change? It doesn't cost much. In fact, if you could reverse the 800 pounds of animal products we consume every year to the fifteen pounds, on an average, it would cost much less, ultimately giving us back huge returns not only in our wallets but by way of recapturing our own precious vital health. Here's an example of how to change your life in ninety days.

Slow and steady wins the race. When you take it slow, the changes you make will be more permanent and natural. Even if you do not use any of our recipes in this book, we decided it would be good to give you a great start by just changing your food choices within this 90 day period. In this way, you can start unwinding an old lifstyle that can be altered easily in these next ninety days and then you may want to add in more and

Going Green in 90Days

Phase I - First month

1. Remove all white (meaning refined) sugars from your diet.
2. Remove all white flour from your diet, including white rice.
3. Remove all fried foods from your diet.
4. Remove 100 percent of all foods that contain unnatural ingredients. (nothing artificial)
5. Remove tap water from your diet completely (even in restaurants).
6. If you drink alcohol at all, give up 25 percent.
7. Remove 25 percent of your coffee drinking.
8. Stop going to all fast-food restaurants.
9. Remove 50 percent soft drink consumptions.
10. Remove 25 percent of your animal consumption, particularly deli meats and pork.
11. Remove 25 percent of all dairy products, except yogurt.Only non-pasteurized yogurt with biffidus/acidophilus cultures added.

Phase II – Second Month

1. Remove all breads which contain yeast / dough conditioners/ mono-diglycerides.
2. Remove 25 percent more of all meats.
3. Remove 25 percent more of alcohol.
4. Remove 25 percent more of coffee drinking.
5. Remove soft drinks entirely .
6. Remove 25 percent more of dairy foods, except yogurt.
7. Find outdoor things to do 10 hours per week.

Phase III – Third Month

1. Remove 25 percent more of all meats.
2. Remove 25 percent more alcohol.
3. Remove 25 percent more coffee drinking.
4. Remove the rest of the dairy eating, except yogurt.

Substitution Foods

1. Add natural sweeteners such as: date sugar, stevia liquid, honey, and rice syrup.
2. Consume only whole grains.
3. Bake or broil foods in place of frying.
4. Consume only bottled or canned foods that contain natural ingredients. (no chemicals or additives)
5. Drink only pure water (steam distilled –we recommend also Evian, Trinity)*
6. Drink 100 percent sugar-free dark grape juice, pomegranate juice, or all berry juice in place of alcoholic drinks
7. Replace coffee drinking with drinks such as: Tecchino, green tea, pero, Sanocafe or other grain coffee substitutes.
8. Find natural food grocery stores that have their own deli, salad bars and juice bars to substitute for fast food eating.
9. Substitute soda drinking for fresh juicing at home. (Carbonation is toxic.)
10. Substitute meat eating with tofu, beans, and various veggie meats.
11. Substitute breads for pita breads, essene breads or whole wheat tortillas.
12. Substitute all dairy products with tofu, soy but keep the unpasteurized yogurt.
13. Take one tablespoon every day of greens such as spirulina or combinations of green powders we recommend. (see Resources)*

14. Substitute all meats with garden burgers, St. Yves Vegetarian meats – they have a huge selection of different types of deli veggie meats, sausages and burgers. They also have vegetarian chicken, which most people swear is almost identical. What makes these products better than animal flesh? First, they are made with

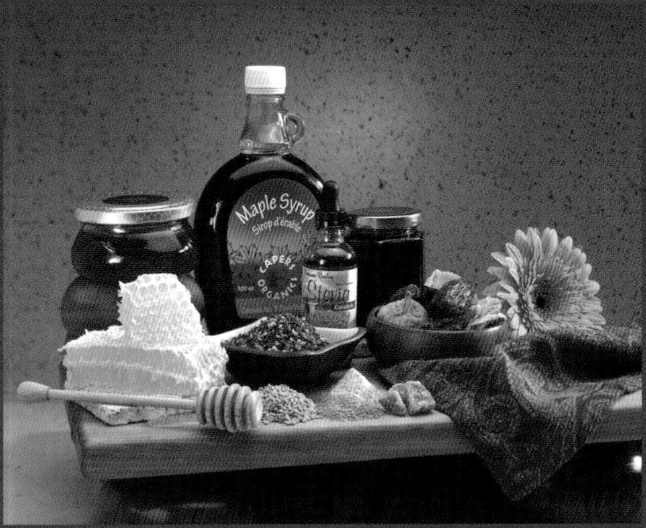

vegetarian proteins from wheat gluten and/or tofu products, a great protein substitute for meats. If you are wheat sensitive or allergic to wheat in any way, we suggest the Gardenburger, and/or vegetarian meats that contain tofu or tempeh as a substitute rather than wheat gluten. Go to: www.healthy-eating.com.

The Gardenburger was created by Paul Wenner, who made the first ever Veggieburger in America that you could purchase in restaurants. Jay and I commend him for his foresight back in 1990 when he first started this company.

Eating a burger made from animal flesh, once you think of it in that light, is quite strange. Mad Cow disease is running rampant throughout the world, and our belief is that it's only a matter of time before we find it happening here in America. What crushes us so deeply is that when an outbreak like this happens, thousands of animals are killed instantly. Thousands and thousands. To Jay and I it's insane, because these are animals bred for our consumption only. Forests are flattened to raise cattle in third world countries, and in our own Country, here in the United States, our water table is 85% dry, and it's all due to feeding and raising cattle, poultry, including pigs and others.

Most Americans just don't know these facts, yet Jay and I feel it's our responsibility to find ways to reach the people with this information., so we can all collectively make a decision to change. This is what is so powerful about working with the written word and television, when properly utilized. By these means, we can change our world, truthfully. You alone can make it happen. Manufacturing companies, including slaughter houses only breed and kill these animals because of the demand. If the demand lessens, cruel killings end and our natural resources are preserved. It's as easy as that.

Our job is only to inform and enlighten. It's up to you to decide whether to act or not.. A plethora of accurate information can be found on the internet. We believe it will change the way you think about a lot of things, including food choices.

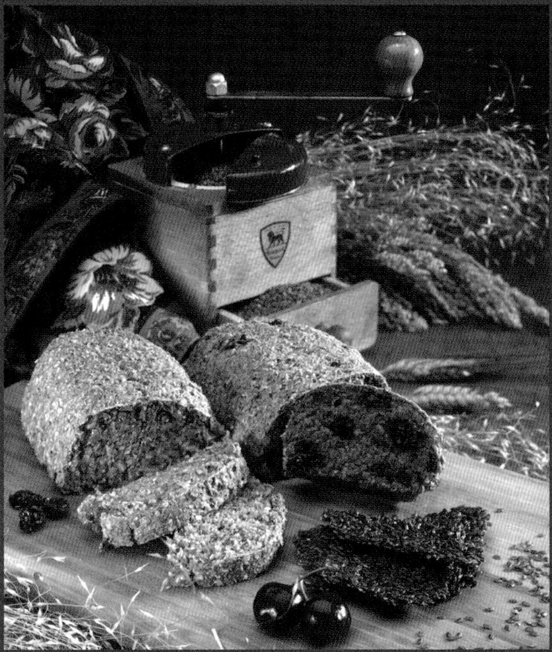

Take the Test – How ALIVE are you?

Taking this test will help you decide which recipes are the best to start with first:

1. How many green* foods do you consume a day?
A. (3) B. (less than 3) or C. (0)
*Green foods, meaning green vegetables, super-green foods, super-green supplements or super-green protein bars, cooked or living green based soups.

2. How much vegetable juice do you drink per day?
A. (32 or more ounces) or B. (less than 32) or C. (0)

3. How much fresh fruit do you eat daily? A. (5 or more) B. (less than 3) C. (0)

4. How much raw (living foods) salads do you eat daily? A. (1/2 -1 lb. or more) B. (less than 1/2 lb) or C. (0).

5. How much do you exercise per day? A. (more than 30 minutes) B. (less than 30) or C. (0).

6. How much water do you consume per day? A. (more than 96 ounces or 2 liters) B. (less than 96 ounces or 2 liters) c. (under 50 ounces or 1.5 liters)

7. How stressed are you? A. (pretty relaxed most of the time) B. (up to 50% stressed) C. (more than 50% stressed)

8. How much animal flesh foods do you consume daily? A. (0) B. (10 oz or less per day) C. (more than 10oz. per day)

9. How much dairy products do you consume daily?
A.(0) B.(10oz. or less) C.(10 oz. or more)

10. Do you smoke? A. (none) B. (less than one pack) C. (more than two packs per day)

11. Do you drink alcohol – including wine or beer?
A. (none) B. (less than two drinks per day) C. (more than two drinks per day)

12. Do you take antacids daily? A. (zero) B. (less than two per day) C. (more than two)

13. Do you have trouble digesting salads?
A. ((hardly ever) B. (Sometimes) C. (Most times)

A = 5 points B=3 points C= 0 points

If you scored between 28-35 points, you can start the transition 1 diet, our mostly 75% living food recipes

If you scored between 17-27 points, you can start the transition 2 diet, our mostly 50% living food recipes

If you scored between 7 – 16 points you can start the transition 3 diet, under 50% living food recipes.

If you scored under 7 points, we highly recommend you see your doctor before considering starting this lifestyle diet change. Since most of us have a lot of toxins build up over the years, sometimes we experience discomforts when we begin to eat a more purifying diet. Symptoms such as digestive disturbances, and/or diarrhea are just really detoxification symptoms, which you will find listed on page 27. For some people it can be uncomfortable because they may have grueling work schedules, therefore the reasons to start slowly. However, most of these symptoms disappear within a week, but is well worth the effort and courage to make this change.

In Chapter 8, you will find three different Live Foods Live Bodies recipes for your new lifestyle. We designed this to make sure you naturally evolve into a lifetime of long-term healthy choices. You will find the transition diet numbers located on each of the recipes. If you start on our Live Foods Live Bodies food program for two weeks, you will be able to move up or down in any direction you like. Usually it's the first two weeks where all the digestive adjustments take place.

Don't Like Greens?

We encourage you to throw out your negative misconceptions about greens and vegetables. Most of us just don't like them, and there may be good reason. Perhaps your parents made you eat your greens and veggies, like Linda's father did. She told me a story once about her childhood. When Linda was about seven years old, she made a big mistake thinking she could outsmart her Dad at the dinner table. He told her one summer evening during dinner, *"If you don't eat your carrots and string beans, you'll sit at this dinner table until midnight, and then some!"* Well, after an hour of sitting, she figured I'd had enough, but he knew if she looked cross-eyed at him, she'd get a whipping, and sure enough it happened. Out went her tongue, glaring at him in defiance and within minutes came the consequence.

To this day, she confesses she could not tolerate cooked carrots until she turned forty! When she married me back in 1981, the KING of carrots, she thought God had punished her. However, she became grateful for the little things in life: Thank God I didn't cook them.

Kids Embracing Vegetables?

If your children do not like cooked vegetables, then we suggest making them vegetable juices,

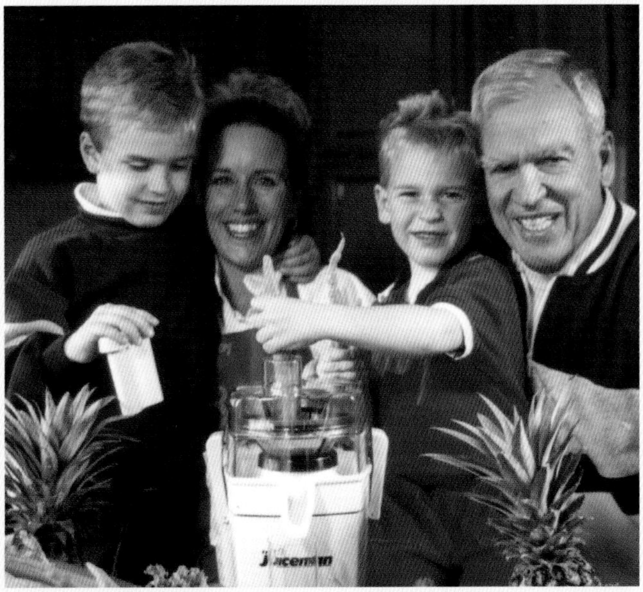

Our kids juicing with us in 1989

combined with a little fresh apple juice. See page 23 for kids recipes. If they don't want to help you make the fresh juice (which is rare), then our suggestion is to put the vegetable juice in a dark glass. Carrot juice is very sweet, and combined with greens, your children will be surprised by how tasty these juices can be. The color, however, can really get them going, thus for the need for a dark glass. This always worked with our children.

So, if you have a horror story like Linda did relating to vegetables, my heart goes out to you, because truthfully no one should ever touch a child in a violent or belligerent way. Children are innocent, period. As far as I'm concerned all children are angels. It's just that sometimes we can't remember back what it's like to be tender, sensitive and vulnerable as all children are. If you become frustrated with your child or grandchild's eating habits, remember; all children really want is to feel safe and be loved. Once we can give them an environment like that, even if we didn't have it ourselves, our children become not only wonderful adults, they become wonderful parents.

I can remember years ago I would lecture to people by saying, "You will start to crave green salads if you can consume them on a daily basis for five to seven days."

For some people it may take up to ten days because once a person starts to consume greens on a daily basis, he will start to detoxify immediately, which can be alarming for some, which is why we push it to ten days at the most. Why? For example, within the first five days, you are getting used to your bowels loosening up more than usual. Some people start to break out in pimples, and some may feel a slight headache for a few days. Some people may feel fantastic, but those are the types of people who have spent longer times eating more pure foods. However, if you are experiencing some negative reactions, be patient, this will pass within a week. If it doesn't, then we suggest you lighten up on

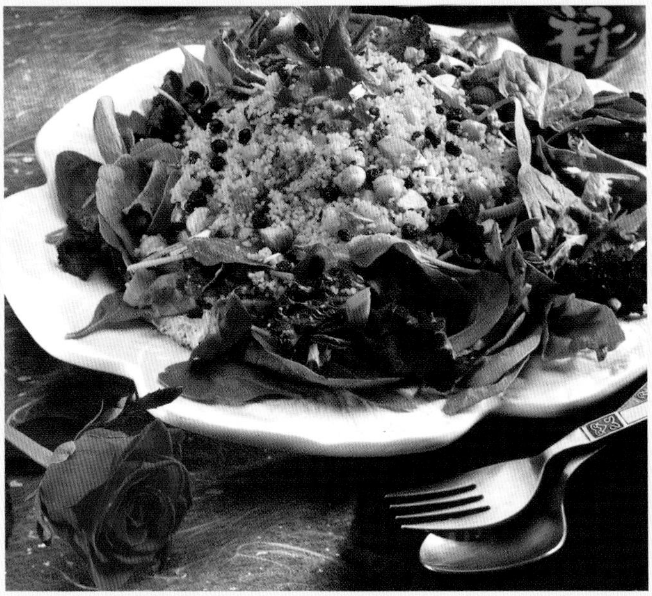

the greens and slow down to only one large whole meal salad per day.

Greens Do Our Bodies Good

There is nothing more wonderful than consuming greens in your daily diet. Here's the payback: beautiful skin, ease of bowel movements, calming nerves, and a more gentle approach to life. Who wouldn't want that? Recent research tells us Americans consume only fifteen pounds or more of greens per year, versus over 800 pounds of animal flesh per year. That would be per person. Alarming, isn't it? In other countries such as Japan and China, this is not the case. Their diets are rich with greens, and especially from the Japanese, greens from the sea such as seaweeds are consumed on a daily basis too. These greens are mineral, vitamin, and phytochemically rich. You will find a recipe we love on page 123 which uses Nori, a seaweed found in most natural food grocery stores in America. Nori is about eight inches square, and is more famously known because it's used to make sushi. Some Nori seaweeds have already been heated, while some are not. If the Nori is green in color, then you will discover this is the type of seaweed that is not cooked. If it is black in color, then it has been toasted. If you are not used to eating Nori, we suggest you eat the toasted kind. The flavor is a bit easier to handle.

Living Greens vs Cooked Greens

Linda and I do not usually eat cooked greens. Let me rephrase that. I never eats cooked greens. Why? Spinach, for example, contains most of its healing properties when eaten or juiced in its living form. When we juice, we do not cook the fruits and vegetables first! This is why juicing has healing qualities. For example, carrot/spinach combined in a format of 60-75 percent carrots and 25-40 percent spinach, you will find that if you consume this combination on and off for a twenty-four hour period, most all stomach ailments cease. That would include diarrhea, constipation, gas, cramping, ulcer-like symptoms, or just a simple stomach ache. When spinach is cooked, it just does not have these kinds of healing properties in them, as all the enzymes are dead, and of course most of the vitamin content has been compromised, including some minerals, thus the reasoning behind Jay not eating cooked greens. For our children and me, steamed broccoli tastes really great in salads, along with other veggies such as green beans.

The only greens we usually cook are greens such as broccoli and a variety of green beans

Why? Broccoli is harder to eat in its uncooked form. However, try steaming it a bit, toss it into a beautiful green salad, and we're in better shape. The same would go for the string beans. Juicing is totally different. Nothing should ever be cooked before juicing, and that would include broccoli and string beans.

If you practice incorporating greens into your life on a daily basis, you will experience waking up in the mornings with ease. Your eyes will not be crusted over, and you will not feel sluggish whatsoever. Your bowels will move properly in the mornings, allowing you tremendous natural energy that will last throughout the day. No coffee will be needed to wake you up, and no alcohol in the evening to bring you down. Further, the addictions to coffee aren't so pronounced, because you're not tired in the morning, nor will you need alcohol to bring you down at night from the caffeine highs from earlier in the day.

Power Up With Super Foods

Super foods play an important role towards a superiordiet.Superfoodsareunrefined,concentrated foods that are taken in small doses to provide highly concentrated doses of nutrients that cannot be compared to any other foods on the planet.

Moreover, these plant-derived foods have been esteemed through the ages. Jay and I use super foods in our power-up drink every single morning, and we highly suggest you start this regime yourself. Our Superfood Smoothie are located on page 183.

Here are some Superfoods we recommend you add into your diet slowly and carefully. Superfoods are full of super-power, so be a bit careful.

Chlorella a green algae that appeared on Earth billions of years ago, is a supplement long popular in Japan and more recently in America. It is valued for its substance named "Chlorella Growth Factor," or CGF. A nucleic acid substance found within each cell, CGF enhances the functions of RNA and DNA in the body by promoting growth and healing. RNA and DNA are responsible for producing protein, enzymes and cellular energy. Since RNA and DNA production slows down with age, chlorella has been shown to benefit our bodies by being one of the richest food sources of RNA and DNA.

It also contains significant amounts of vitamins B-12 and A and is rich in chlorophyll. Chlorophyll is the green pigment in growing plants that is similar to human blood in chemical structure. Chlorophyll has been shown to increase our red blood cell count. This capability can lead to better oxygenation of cells, resulting in improved body cleansing because cell waste is then removed more quickly. Chlorella is typically ingested in pressed tablet form.

Green Barley comes from barley grass and, like chlorella, is high in chlorophyll and valued since biblical times. It is rich in magnesium, potassium, beta-carotene and vitamin C. While it is often used to relieve colds and flu, research has demonstrated its effectiveness in treating skin disorders, protecting against radiation, repairing damaged cells, and in treating chronic diseases of the pancreas.

Green barley comes in powder or tablet form. The young leaves of green barley are either juiced and dehydrated or milled into a powder. The powder can be dissolved in cool water, milk or juice. It's best to start with a small amount of green barley because some people develop diarrhea with regular doses. Others develop constipation when taking Green Barley Essence because it is low in fiber. To avoid this, simply eat vegetables at the same time.

Wheatgrass is actually young wheat plants. When only a few inches in height, the tender blades can be juiced or turned into tablets, pellets or powder. Wheat grass is high in chlorophyll, pro-vitamin A, vitamins B, C, and E, and is a good source of calcium, potassium, magnesium, selenium and zinc. It contains some iron. We think it best to drink the fresh juice rather than eat dehydrated forms since juice is easily assimilated without losing its nutrients.

Spirulina

Spirulina is a blue-green micro algae, a tiny aquatic plant that can be seen only through a microscope. Spirulina's introduction as a supplement in America was in 1979, but its existence dates to the beginning of plant life on Earth. Spirulina's significance as a food source lies in its being 60 percent to 70 percent protein by weight, which is twice the amount that of dried milk and almost one-third more than whole dried eggs or brewer's yeast.

This concentrated food contains high amounts of vitamin B-12 and other B vitamins. Also present are biotin, pantothenic acid, folic acid and inositol. The concentrated presence of gamma-linolenic acid (GLA) has been shown to help degenerative diseases like arthritis and heart disease. It is not promoted as a weight loss aid, but people using spirulina before meals report having greater control over their food intake.

Bee Pollen pollen is the male germ seed produced by all flowering plants. Bees use this seed for their protein source and deposit the seed in waxy cells. Pollen, like spirulina, is a rich source of protein—about 23 percent by weight. It is low in fat and sodium. It is a good source of pro-vitamin A, the B vitamins except B-12, calcium, magnesium and zinc. It has a moderate amount of vitamin C as well.

Pollen is known to help problems of the prostate. While pollen comes in tablets, pellets and granules, the best type is fresh pollen granules from your local beekeeper. That way you know the pollen has been collected by bees in a toxic-free locale. When this is not possible, using pollen pellets is best. Be sure to store fresh pollen in the refrigerator. It is best to always purchase bee pollen in organic form.

Below you will find a quick-start approach to getting greens into your body without too much struggle:

Get Your (Uncooked) Greens Fast

Here is a quick-start approach toward getting your superfoods into your daily diet:

- Fresh vegetable juices
- Powdered greens sprinkled over salads or into juices
- Smoothies · Super salads · Living soups

Frustrated?

Remember not to be too hard on yourself. If you find yourself craving sweets, then by all means, try satisfying yourself with a few dates. If you're the kind of person that one bite makes fifty more, then I suggest you stay without anything sweet for at least ten days, as your tastes buds will gradually change. Dates are very sweet, yet very good for you. Try one of our recipes on page 179. These smoothies are sweet enough to squelch any cravings, within reason, of course.

How to Get UnAddicted from Fast Foods-FAST

As I said in an earlier chapter, Jay has a more male approach by saying, to heck with fear and frustration, "just do it!" I say, let's slow down a bit and take a longer look at our predicament. For example, if you are overweight, stressed out, lethargic, bloated from too much consumption of sugar or salt and packaged foods, yet inside of you is a person dying to come out that does not look like the person staring back at you in the mirror, then I would say, it's not just your food habits that are betraying you. There's a lot more to this struggle than is visible to the naked eye. Addiction and denial could be the problem.

Certain foods ARE addictive. This is a real problem in America today. Why? Food manufacturers know this and capitalize on this factor. Their number one goal is to please their stockholders and to keep their jobs. Their main objective is to profit the company, not to make you healthy! It's a travesty, in my opinion, but once you realize you don't HAVE to be on their agenda, that indeed you can create your own agenda, completely free from their lair so to speak. You CAN be free to be exactly what you want, eat what your want and when you want it, but not before you learn how to empower yourself with the foods that can literally change your life in as little as a week.

Here's what you need to do immediately to stop the addiction to the foods that are controlling your life::

◆ Quit eating or drinking sugar of all kinds for ten days.

◆•Quit consumption of all flours for ten days.

◆•Get off stimulants such as coffee, black tea or green teas.

◆•Stop eating all meats, including fish.

◆·Do not drink any kind of alcohol.*

◆•Do not smoke cigarettes or marijuana or take any kind of non-prescription mind altering drugs, unless your doctor has prescribed them specifically for you.

Here's What You can Do in Place:

◆ Exercise thirty minutes per day, even if it's just gardening in the sun.

◆ Drink approximately 100 ounces of steam-distilled water throughout the day.

◆·Eat any of our recipes in this book, except for the deserts (for the first ten days).

◆ Drink any amount of herbal teas desired without sweeteners.

◆ Try to consume one super-green smoothie per day.

◆ Try to get sun every day for at least 30 minutes. If you work, take a walk during lunch break. Use this time to calm your mind, unwind, and connect with nature.

◆Take enzyme and probiotic supplementation during these first ten days with every meal.

◆ Drink at least one quart of vegetable juices daily with a ratio of 25 percent greens such as spinach, parsley, kale, endive, escarole, romaine lettuce, baby field greens. If you are interested in wheat grass juice, take only with foods during the first ten days, as the wheat grass has a very strong detoxification factor to it. When you consume it with foods, it will ease into the bloodstream at a slower rate, making it easier for your body to assimilate .

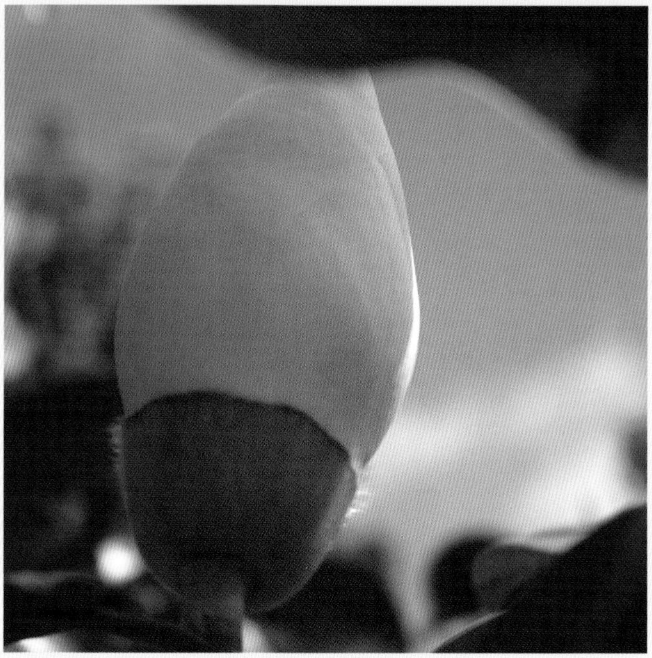

Lose Weight = Feel Great = Freedom

Here's the good news: Not only will you feel a tremendous amount of freedom from the addiction to the foods you used to eat, but you will lose weight, too! Most people lose around five to ten pounds during the first ten days eating this way. If you drink coffee in the mornings, I can assure you, you will drink alcohol in the evenings. We pike ourselves up in the mornings so high, that we need another drug to bring us down in the evenings. That would be alcohol. Thus starts the vicious circle going. Cigarette smoking falls somewhere in between these two vices. So, if you just cannot stop smoking all at once (which we know is very hard to do), then we suggest you try to do all of the above except the smoking, and keep it as low as possible. Within time, the smoking will take a more passive role in your life with enough distraction and commitment to eating and living a more natural and fulfilled lifestyle. Once you start to remove the alcohol and coffee, the smoking takes on an entire new reality, thus enabling you to quit faster and most important – permanently. One of the main reasons people don't like to break addictions is because it brings up huge emotional issues that need to be cleared if we are to clear the addiction. Finding a good therapist who concentrates on Bach Flower Essence therapy is a wonderful approach to healing all addictions. (See Web site and Resources).

Frankly, it takes approximately three full months of eating this way to feel confident you will not go back to the addictive behavior. The good news is that if indeed you slip up, you are now ***empowered*** with the knowledge that these can heal you and support vital health. Jay and I recommend you take the following supplements along with the living food and super foods you will be incorporating into your diet: calcium/magnesium supplements, Co-enzyme Q10, Grapeseed extract, full spectrum amino acids, Vitamin C from Camu/Camu berries, Omega 3 oils, Bach Flower Remedies. (See Web sites and Resources for Bach Flower Remedies).

How Got Well
How You Can get Well (Linda)

Unfortunately, I came from a background filled with emotional and psychological abuse during my teenage years, including being abandoned whereby I ended up becoming a slave to anorexia and bulimia by the time I reached eighteen. In 1974 nobody ever heard of annorexia/bulemia until Cherry Boone wrote the book, Starving for Attention back in 1976.

My entire life became a dark hell for almost nine years. I finally realized as I crawled out of the hell I was living in for so long, that correct food choices would not heal my heart and soul entirely. Changing behaviors, seeing the dark side to the illness, surrendering to a greater power than myself for healing, were some of the first things I started to acknowledge and incorporate before I started to get well. Unfortunately, it wasn't until I was very ill that I started to connect the dots, finally understanding annorexia/bulemia was not about food. This mystery took many years to understand.

Food addictions are Not About Foods

Even if you are not addicted to foods or do not have an eating disorder, you can definitely benefit from what I did to get well, as only eight years ago, Jay and I suffered a severe loss in our lives that turned our *entire* world upside down. One of the first things we did was to re-create the steps shown below to help our souls heal from the devastation we endured. This process we are about to show you is also good for overcoming grief, loss, divorce, abandonment, betrayals, loss of job, personal identity, bankruptcy, emotional trauma or long term illness.

As I've said earlier, it's not just pure food that will heal us from our ill health. Our minds are much more powerful than we realize. Our minds can liberate us, or they can destroy us. Only you can be the master of your own mind. The best way to master our mind is to start a form of discipline described on the next page.

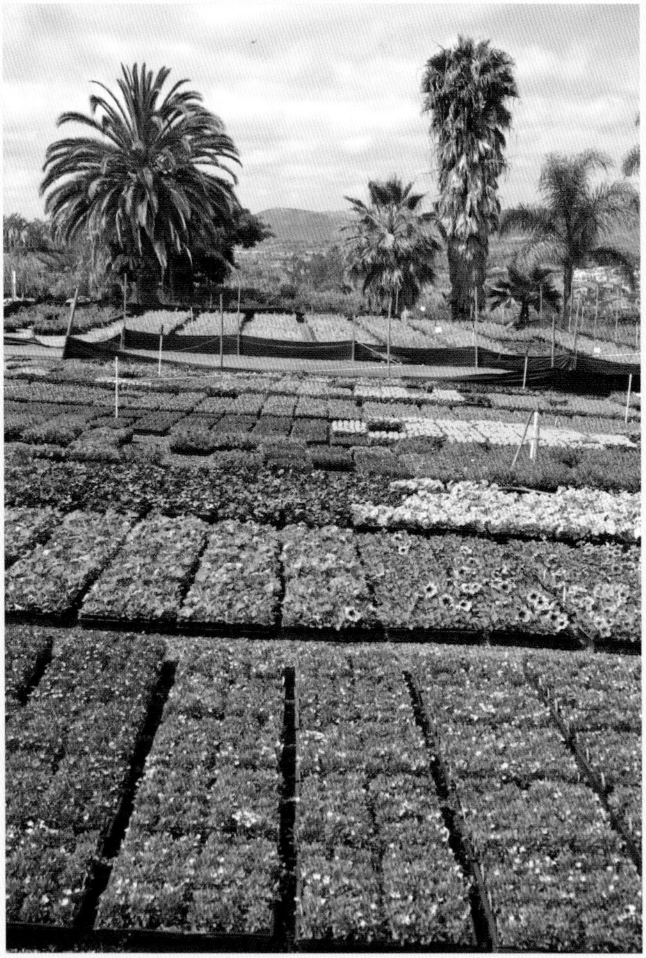

Here's what we did for approximately 90 days to focus on our health, heal our hearts and souls, and most importantly, to reconnect to God and nature:

◆Turn off television for 30 days.(read the paper)

◆Cut out all socializing with negative people 100%

◆ Spend at least 2 hours outside in a garden daily.*

◆Read autobiographical materials that inspires you

◆Do not go out at nights, or weekends, unless it is to get produce or go to church, or to help others or listen to lectures that are uplifting.

◆Dry-brush massage your skin for ten minutes before bath time.

◆Drink up to two quarts of vegetable juices daily, throughout the day, carrot combined mostly with 30-50 percent greens: parsley,spinach,kale,broccoli, endive,wheatgrass.(see digestive juice aids on page 20-21)

◆Drink up to 100 ounces of pure water daily (preferably steamed distilled water).

◆Make evenings sacred: Take long baths with lavender oil before bedtime if you're a woman. If you're a man, we suggest saunas or steam baths at a gym either after work or after dinner.

◆Listen to inspiring music during meals, or in the evenings before bedtime (for example: Yanni, Enya, yoga meditation and/or classical).

◆Exercise daily for at least thirty minutes.

◆Take one hour-long walk every night before sun down, or in the morning.

◆Meditate or pray for grace and/or peace and understanding for thirty minutes per day, either early in morning or before bedtime.

◆ Write down every emotion you have—who you have issues, who you love, appreciate and who you are grateful for, who you admire, what you wanted to become-how you need to change, and who you need to forgive so you can be free**

◆Only consume living foods or only fruits, seeds, nuts, vegetables, herbs, berries and grains.

Create a sacred living space for yourself in the kitchen (for example, we put a picture of our family and our beautiful dog, Simba, next to it, too. We then light a candle and asked God to protect our family and to bless the foods prepared.)

*If you do not have a food garden or a flower garden, we suggest you find a community garden to work in as much as you can.

***Forgiveness was the most important step we made, now that we look back at our life. We had a lot of emotional trauma that kept us from living in the present, which is crucial to creating a future life. Journaling every night was also a wonderful experience for me. Journaling can be a cathartic outlet to connect to that part of yourself that rarely gets heard.*

Extra Tips

If you work full time, believe me, you can still do these exercises mentioned above. If you have some vacation time coming, then use it for something like this. It's doesn't cost a penny. Invest in yourself. Remember simplicity? The simple life is the best life!

If you work full time, what I recommend is that you do the exercises in the evenings, and skip the walking. The sacred bath time can be worked out after you get home from work.

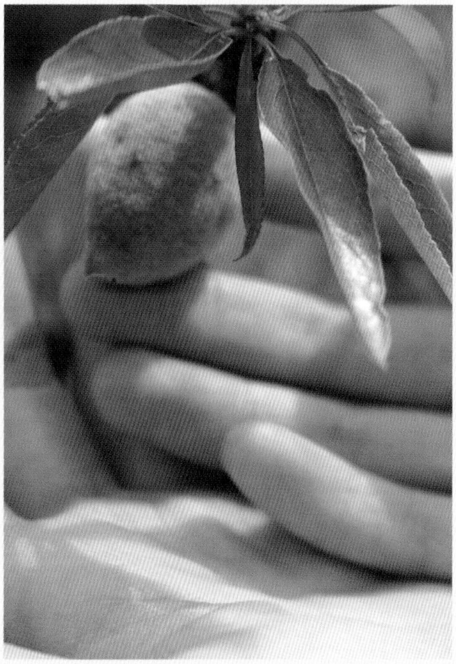

Enlist your spouse to do the meals for the children, while you concentrate on yourself. If he won't do it, or if you are single, then it's ok. It will still work. Garden time of two hours per day can be mostly used up during the weekends. Journaling can also easily be incorporated early mornings or in the evenings during your sacred bath time.

The reasons I recommend so much outdoor time is because part of getting well, as I said earlier is that

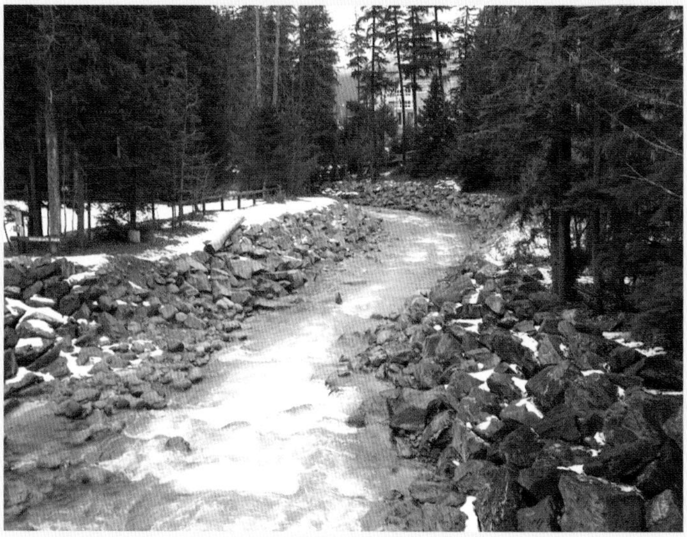

it's not just all about foods, it's about our relationship with the world and the relationship we have with ourselves. The sun gives us a tremendous amount of vital energy, and what I love to call - Solar Love. It's true! When we spend time in the sun, whatever is bothering us seems to diminish. Even our skin needs the sun. Our pituitary gland needs the sun to covert Vitamin D into our bodies. Jay talks about the sun in more depth in his tape, How To Live To Be 100-Disease Free. You can find it on our Web site: www.jaykordich.com. You will learn about why it's so important to be in the sun every day.

Gratitude is our Greatest Liberator

When I was ill during my late teens and early twenties trying to survive an eating disorder, I discovered that I started to heal myself by loosing myself through creating delicious meals, juices and smoothies for those I loved. This included my neighbors, business contacts and anyone who needed my help, that within enough time, and using nature to help guide and heal me, this devastating disorder eventually disappeared from my life as strangely as it appeared. If you have not suffered an addiction to foods, but are basically frustrated and depressed in life, trust me; serving others is the key to liberation. You may not want to hear this, but it's true. It's one of those universal truths we cannot ignore. Find a way to serve your children, your community your parents, grandchildren or your spouse, without any need for gain or merit. It will take time. Here's the truth: When you serve others without any desire for merit or gain, you are ultimately serving yourself. This is where the healing comes into play.

So, for me, I found my authentic self through serving others, and by listening to that quiet voice of God, guiding me to do the right thing. Once incorporated, simplicity naturally created the balance and joy I so desired and needed in my life, thus the release from the addiction slowly disappeared.

I will leave you with an interesting concept someone shared with me about ten years ago, that still intrigues me today:

A large tree will only sense your presence if you sit still, under the tree and not move for five days. It will only then see you for an instant. Amazing isn't it? We go so fast in life. We miss so much. When we learn to slow down, not only will we discover so much more to nature and natural foods and natural living, we may discover a person you haven't seen since childhood—yourself!

We hope this chapter has opened a door for you to see there is future and hope, knowing our health is our greatest wealth, free to all, yet all we have to do is to learn from those who have tread the path, incorporate this knowledge and instill some discipline into our lives, and *know* this is your heritage, free to all who desire it. We can all be well, balanced and especially empowered with the knowledge natural foods has to give us, which is a future without the fear of hospitalizations, drugs, depression, frustration and despair.

Don't you think it's worth a try? If you have any questions, please don't hesitate to reach us. Jay and I extend our deepest gratitude to you for your support, and wish you the vital health awaiting you, and for all those who you love. But first, let's find out about the mysteries of enzymes, and how they will play an important role in your near future as you work towards a diet rich in living foods..

“Enzymes are Life’s

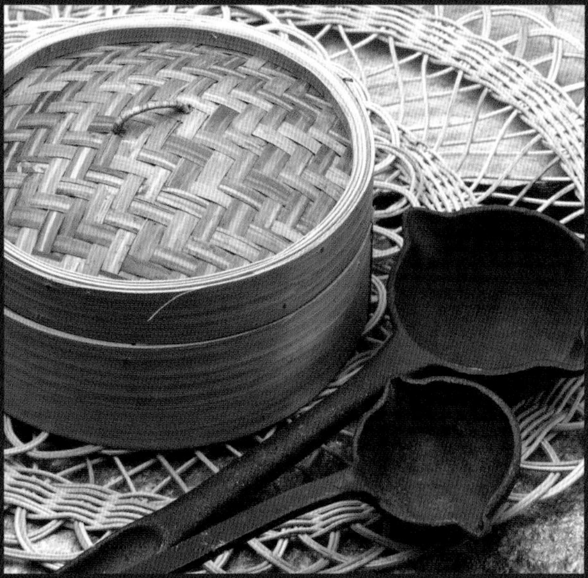

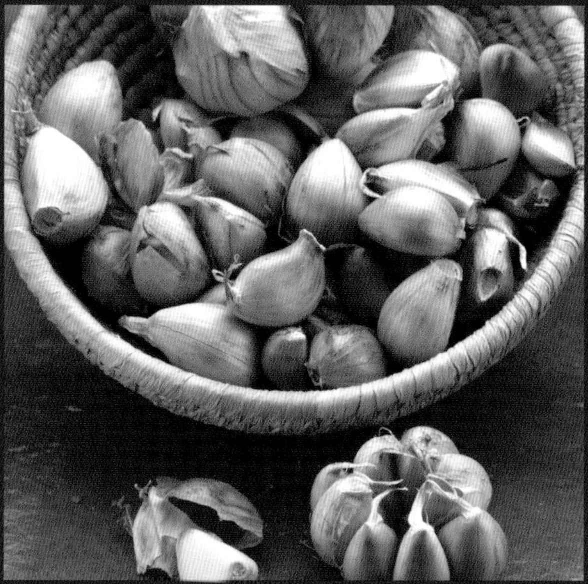

"Fountain of Youth"

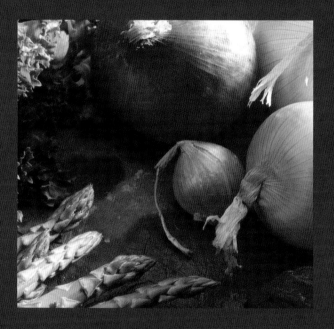

-Jay Kordich

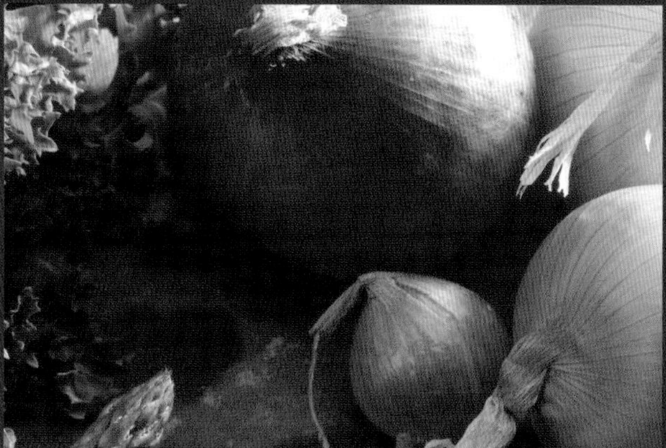

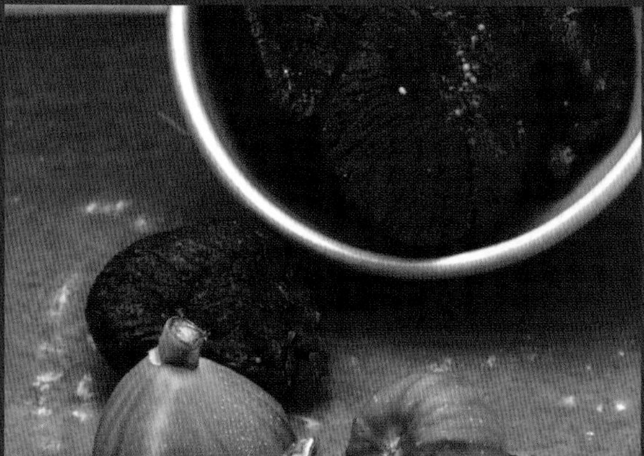

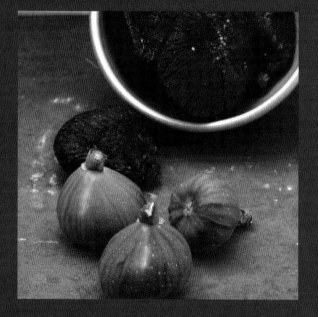

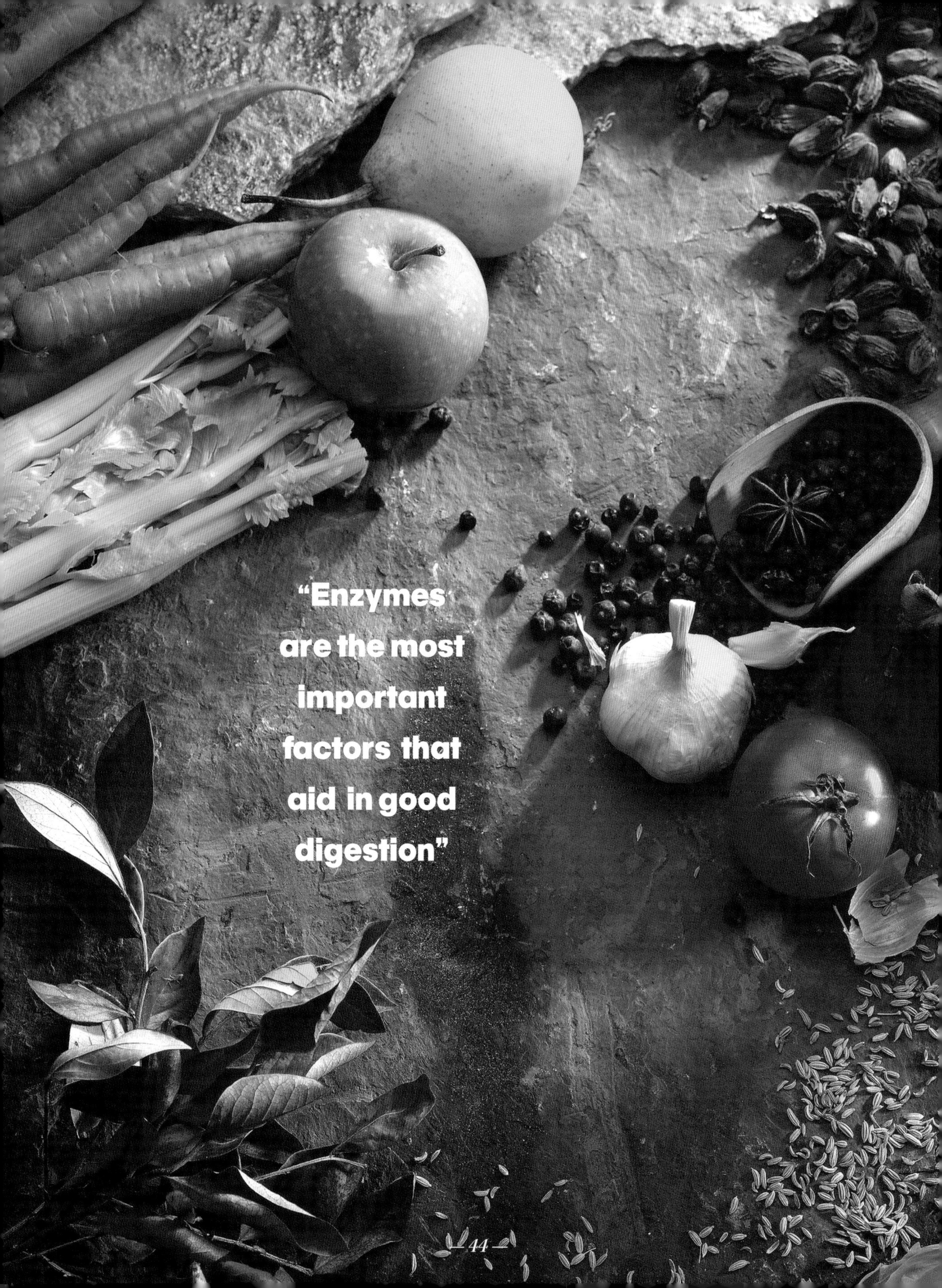

"Enzymes are the most important factors that aid in good digestion"

Chapter 4
Enzymes Equal Energy

- Why Plant Enzymes are so Important to our Diet
- How to Build you own "Enzyme Bank Account"
- How to Make cooked food 'Come Alive'.
- Twelve Easy Steps for more natural Enzyme Power

The Secret Key to Vitality

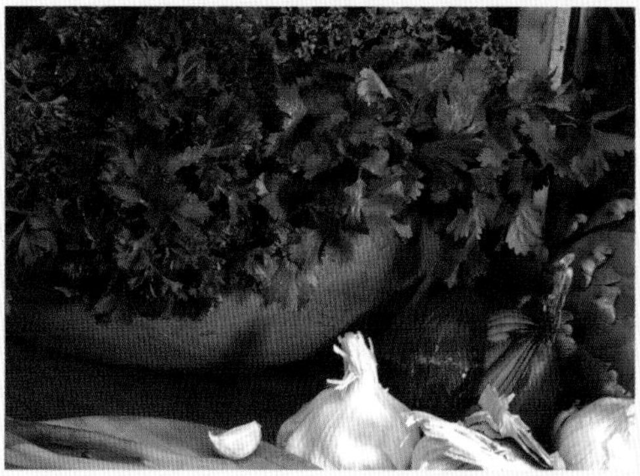

The key to vitality is simple. it lies within plant enzymes! The difference between live, living, sun-baked foods and cooked, devitalized foods is the presence or lack of enzymes. It is known that cooking foods, even placing them in boiling water, virtually kills all enzymes. Baking bread kills enzymes. Most dairy products don't have enzymes. However, if you read a label of cheese at the grocery store, it will say it contains enzymes. These are not the enzymes we are talking about. This reference to enzymes is the cow intestine used to help coagulate and form the cheese. (hard to believe, but true) Most dairy products don't have any natural enzymes, because most dairy products are pasteurized. Juices sold in cartons, cans and bottles may have some vitamins and minerals, but you can be assured the enzymes are long gone. A diet composed of all (or mostly) cooked devitalized foods deprives the body of the enzyme nutrition it needs to properly function day in and day out. It is surprising—even alarming— that more people do not understand this basic biological fact. Yet, where have we read different? The story of the importance of enzymes in our diets is just recently being discovered.

Plant Enzymes Live Only in Raw Foods

Enzymes, in the human body, work as catalysts and in that role are key to the workings of the entire body. Enzyme activity begins from the moment an egg is fertilized by sperm, and it does not stop until the day we die. Enzymes initiate, direct or accelerate virtually every chemical reaction required for life. Absolutely nothing happens without enzymes. Breathing, blinking, hearing, smelling, seeing are all are governed by catalytic enzyme activity. Enzymes are required to eat, digest and absorb all nutrients. The immune system depends on enzymes to direct its functions. Enzymes are used by the heart, liver, kidneys, and lungs. Indeed, if it were not for enzymes, your body would be no more than a lifeless pile of chemicals.

Cooking Destroys Fiber-Rich Foods

In addition to enzymes, vegetables and fruits contribute much-needed fiber to our body. When food is eaten in a living and unprocessed state, its fibers act as an intestinal broom to maintain intestinal cleanliness. High-heat cooking destroys the fibrous life in food. The fibers lose their magnetism through the heating process and become devitalized. They now act more like a mop than a broom, swabbing through the intestines, all too often leaving a coating of slime on intestinal walls. In time, this slime accumulates and putrefies, ultimately causing toxemia. The colon then becomes sluggish, causing constipation, colitis, diverticulosis and other disturbances to occur.

For those of you who have colon trouble or challenges, we suggest a thirty-day colon cleanse. Cleanses can really help with better absorption of the foods you eat. Linda and I recommend Dr. Richard Anderson's work. He has written wonderful books on colon health. You can reach his web site, www.ariseandshine.com You may want to speak with your

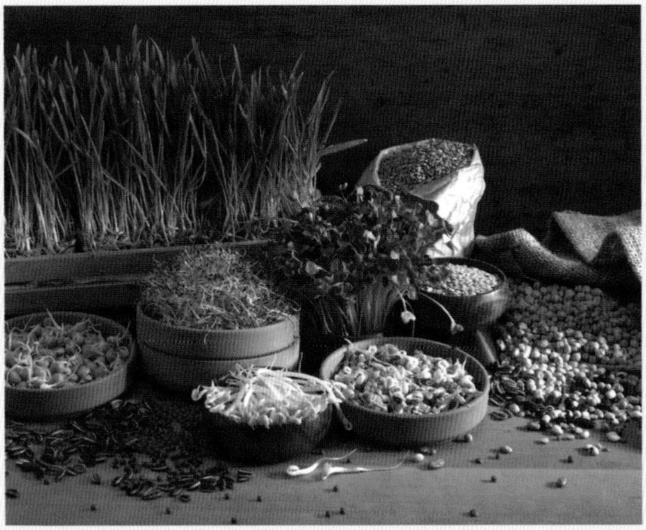

doctor before starting any kind of fast or deep cleanse.

As Doctor Norman Walker, my mentor since 1948, says, "We describe enzymes as an intangible, magnetic, Cosmic Energy of Life Principle, which is intimately involved in the action and activity of every atom in the human body, in vegetation and in every form of life. He continues: "Enzymes are sensitive to temperatures above 118 degrees F. Above 120, enzymes become sluggish, just as the human body becomes languid and relaxed in a hot bath. At 130 F the life of enzymes is extinct. They are dead."

Scientists are Just Discovering the Powers of Food Enzymes

To date, science has identified roughly 3,200 enzymes—and that is likely just the tip of the iceberg. One enzyme helps to build phosphorus in bone. Another causes muscles to contract. Yet another is responsible for the clotting mechanism in blood. Fear, hunger, and sexual arousal are all controlled in the brain by other powerful enzymes. Undeniably, the importance of enzymes is enormous, for enzymes embody the mysterious "life principle," the very energy upon which every living thing thrives. This is why we named our book *Live Foods Live Bodies.* When we consume mostly living foods, our bodies are more alive, our cells thoroughly bathed with living enzymes.

Your natural Enzymes Bank Account

We are all born with a fixed amount of enzymes, a kind of personal enzyme bank account. Those who exist on an enzyme-less diet of cooked, denatured, processed foods wantonly spend their body's precious enzyme reserves. On the other hand, those who regularly consume fresh juices and living juices—which are loaded with enzymes—make regular deposits into their body's enzyme bank account, and thereby avoid unnecessary disease and premature aging.

One of the first to prove the necessity of living food enzymes in human nutrition, respected authority Dr. Edward Howell, put more than 40 years of his life into enzymology research. Two other wonderful doctors we recommend in the enzymology field are Dr. Gabriel Cousins, Spiritual Nutrition, and Dr. Humberto Santillo. They both have written remarkable books, which can be found in chapter 9, under Web sites and Resources. What Dr. Howell discovered in his studies is scientific fact. As we start to find out more and more about enzymes, Dr. Howell's research finds new meaning with experts.

Plant Enzyme Information you Should know About:

Enzymes, present in all living foods, are routinely destroyed by cooking anything over 120 degrees Fahrenheit.
A diet of cooked, refined, enzyme less foods forces the pancreas to work overtime, cranking out extra enzymes in order to process the denatured and devitalized foods and move it through the digestive tract.
This overburdening of the pancreas causes it to become enlarged,just as an overburdened heart muscle enlarges. This results in accelerated aging, an increase in chronic degenerative diseases, and, ultimately, cancer.

When the pancreas is overburdened with regular consumption of enzyme-less food, it is deterred from its function of producing insulin and creating pancreatic enzymes to keep tropoblastic (precancerous) cells at bay. The pancreatic enzymes devour weakened, ailing, even cancerous cells that, left unchecked, may result in all sorts of insidious digestive ailments, such as leaky gut syndrome, acid relfux and colitis.

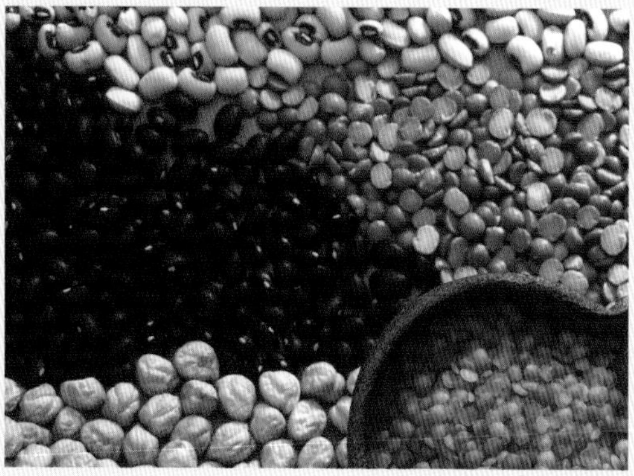

Plant Enzymes to the Rescue

The obvious question is: can we consume more enzymes to improve our health? The answer is an emphatic YES—in the form of living, sun-baked, uncooked, raw foods, and their fresh juices.

You see, all natural foods consumed raw are bursting with enzymes required for their digestion. These food enzymes aren't lazy. They work day and night to break down and digest the millions of cells in the plants we eat, whether they are fruits, vegetables, or herbs. Fresh pineapple, for example, contains the powerful enzyme bromelain; bananas have the enzyme amylase; and papaya, the enzyme papain. Likewise, when you eat a raw carrot, the naturally occurring enzyme it contains does much of the work, breaking that carrot down in your stomach and small intestine.

But juice that carrot and you "do your body good." Freshly prepared juices are essentially predigested food, with nearly all the nutrients—and live enzymes—synergistically intact. Juice a carrot, and you give your body an automatic "enzyme boost," an extra shot of live, usable enzymes ready to go to work for all your vital organs and tissues. This is why we recommend you consume the Digestive Juice Specials (located on page 20-21) with your meals. These juices are rich in enzymes, and if, by chance, you are eating a meal that is not at least 75 percent living, these juices are designed to help digest your cooked meal. It bears repeating from our introduction: Whenever you eat a meal, ask yourself, ***"How much of my meal is alive (meaning enzyme-rich)?"*** This simply means how much raw food in on my plate? This awareness will ultimately change the way you look and feel about foods forever.

Your personal lifestyle and higher-attuned consciousness will determine how far and how quickly you can go with this program. Those living in a warm climate year-round or a more sublime manner of living may find it easier to adapt readily to a new eating routine, while those who are used to fast food, heavy coffee/alcohol consumption and an on-the-go mentality may need to make more moderate changes. Ironically, when we do consume at least 75 percent of our foods from live plant life, nuts, seeds, herbs, and soaked grains, our lives become much more relaxed and balanced.

For those who are not consuming at least 75 percent of their foods in this way, we suggest you consume up to one quart of vegetable juices daily or supplement your diet with enzymes with each meal. You can also add to your cooked meal one of the following: chopped raw onions, chives, or uncooked, fresh, crushed garlic. Adding these items to cooked food helps to make them more "alive" with available natural enzymes for better digestion. We believe the compounds in raw onions and garlic help destroy foreign bacteria and parasitses. Raw onions and garlic contain a natural antiseptic that also helps keep the colon clean.

Enzymes Fight Old Age

As you are beginning to realize, enzymes are essential for the digestion of food and the release of nutrients in the body. The food you eat must first be broken down by enzymes to simpler building blocks and reformulated in the body according to need. The building blocks are used to restore the older, worn-out cells in every part of the body. It is a known fact that the body completely regenerates on a cellular level every seven years, with the exception of part of the brain.

If enzymes are not present in the food, the body cannot digest properly or extract essential nutrients. This leaves the body nutrient-deprived and starved. Without these vital nutrients, the body cannot replace old, dying cells with new cellular growth. Typically, the younger you are, the greater your enzyme reserves. This is why younger people can tolerate a diet of white bread, starches, sugars, animal products, and predominantly cooked foods. Over the years, however, as enzyme reserves decrease, these same foods cause illnesses such as constipation, bleeding ulcers, bloating, and digestive troubles as mentioned before such as leaky gut, colitis, and arthritis. These conditions are only symptoms of intestinal toxemia.

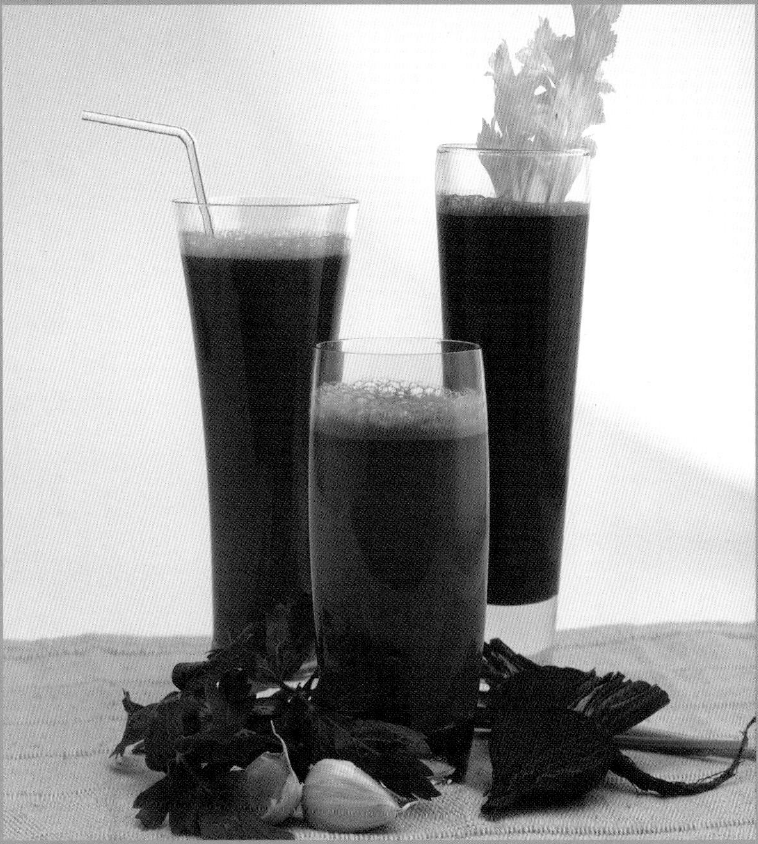

Keep Your Diet Rich with Enzymes

There is still so much to learn about enzymes. Perhaps vitamins and minerals are better absorbed in our bodies when enzymes are present. Perhaps a diet rich in enzymes can help us live to be over 100 years, disease free. We are thrilled that more and more wonderful research is coming out about the miracles of food enzymes. My diet, since 1948, has been rich with enzymes. Luckily, I met a doctor who was worlds ahead of his time, instinctively knowing enzymes were a major key to longevity. I referred to Dr. Max Gerson earlier in chapter 1. The Gerson Clinic, now located in Bonita, California, does impressive work in the field of healing cancer , degenerative diseases, and treating terminally ill people. What saddens me is most Americans don't see that this kind of therapy is so transformative.

Jay's Quick Tips for Better Digestion:

1. Drink a glass of freshly made vegetable juice (see our digestive juice recipes (in Chapter 2)with your cooked or even semi-cooked, and sip it when you are slowly chewing your foods.

2. Make sure to soak your grains, beans and nuts two hours ahead of time, almonds 12 hours before you use them. Macadamia nuts should not be soaked. (If you forget, don't worry, even an hour helps a lot.) Then make sure to rinse them before cooking. Doing this releases an enzyme inhibitor to make these foods much more digestible.

3. Before dinner time, light a candle before you start to prepare your meal. Either say your own affirmation for tranquility and divine guidance, or feel welcome to use ours on page 87. Relaxing like this is wonderful for digestion.

4. If you are eating more than 25 percent of your meal cooked, try chopping up either raw onions or fresh garlic and sprinkle them over your foods to help better digest your meal by adding in more antiseptic foods such as these.

5. If you cannot do steps #1 or #4, take a few digestive enzymes with your meal. You can find our enzymes on our web site.

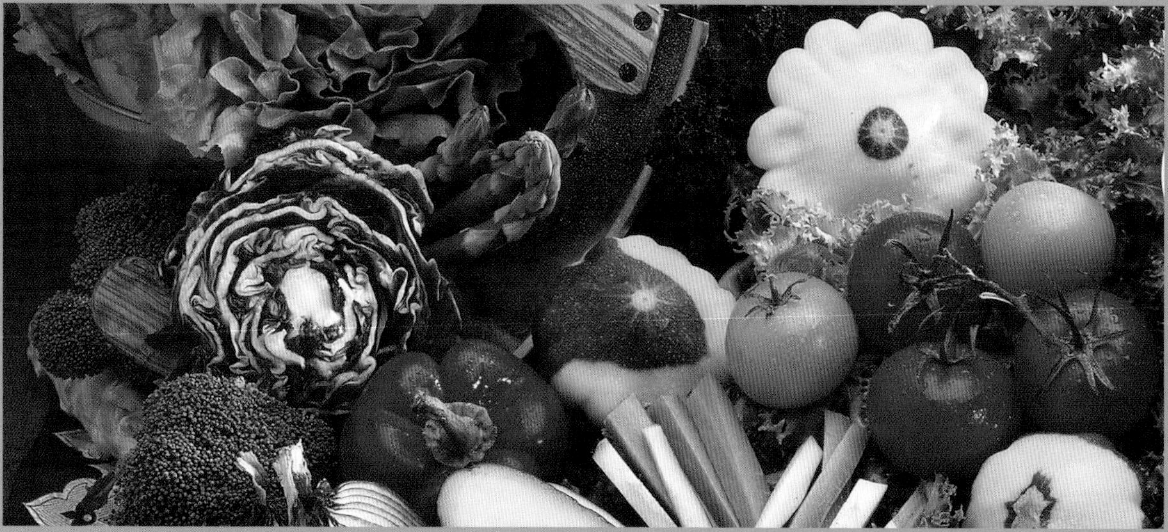

Enzymes are the powerful life catalyst behind every function that the human body performs. They can keep you young, keep you healthy, keep you full of vital energy—even keep you slender (because you are actually metabolizing your food properly), but they need a proper environment to function at their very best. The twelve steps below will help you speedily multiply your body's enzyme reserves, while maximizing its youthful, healthful, life giving benefits.

12 Steps to Maximize

1	**BEGIN** each day with fresh, ripe fruit in season, or your favorite fresh juice combination. My favorite is pineapple/grapefruit, which packs a real enzyme power punch. Most Americans can get pineapple and grapefruits year round. Remember to always peel the grapefruit before juicing, and try to leave as much of the white pulp on the grapefruit as possible. Starting the day with fresh fruit showers your digestive system with enzymes.
2	**LATER**, have something living: a predominately vegetable-based salad with a glass of carrot/spinach juice. If your salad contains any cooked foods, the juice you drink will give your body the enzymes it needs.
3	**DON'T** mix fruits and vegetables in juices, or in your meals, because the enzymes are incompatible and may cause gastric distress. Apples are the exception to this rule. They are enzymatically compatible with either fruits or vegetables. We cover this issue in more detail in chapter 4.
4	**RESTRICT** the amounts of liquids with meals. Too much liquid consumed at mealtime can actually "drown" enzymes, both diluting their power in the stomach and inhibiting their catalytic actions. Drink freely between meals but not sooner than fifteen minutes before or after meals. However, it is acceptable to drink with meals our Digestive Juice Aids discussed in chapter 2.
5	**RESTRICT** your intake of cooked foods (anything cooked over 119 degrees Fahrenheit). If you must cook, the best method is steaming or baking. Avoid fried foods at all costs, and this includes stir frying vegetables.
6	**DRINK** natural beverages, preferably freshly made juices. Avoid coffee, alcohol, cola/carbonated drinks of any kind, and artificial beverages. Caffeine and alcohol destroy digestive juices and enzyme generation. However, organic herbal, green, white, and black teas are recommended. Green and black teas have small amounts of caffeine; however, their high antioxidant power overrides any negative caffeine impact. Tecchino, Caffix and Pero are coffee substitutes made from barley and other grains, which we recommend. Soymilk, rice milk, and almond milk (freshly made) are acceptable. Any of these beverages we have recommended go well with organic honey. We drink plenty of water and usually only steam-distilled, available from most home delivery water companies. If this is unavailable to you, we recommend using reverse osmosis. If you buy water from the store, we only recommend Trinity Springs Water. Never drink tap water, since it contains too many harsh contaminants, resulting, we believe, in kidney stones. Restaurants are notorious for serving tap water. Please make sure to ask your server if they provide filtered water, even in beverages such as tea.

Your Enzyme Power

7	**AVOID** refined sugar. It interferes with healthy metabolism and hinders enzyme activity. What's more, it actually contributes to heart disease. Use organic raw honey instead, since it is full of powerful enzymes. We also recommend Stevia as a sugar substitute, which can be found in either granular or liquid form. Another sugar substitute we recommend is Sucanant, found in the same way.
8	**DON'T** eat cooked foods late at night! Your body is happiest getting this rest period to conduct its internal cleansing and repairs. If you tie up precious enzymes for late-night digestion, your body won't get the rest and recuperation it needs. Please don't make the body work most of the night digesting cooked food. You're much better off retiring with a cup of herbal tea or a calming glass of enzyme rich apple-celery juice. When in season, we love to eat ripe pears in the evening, if we become hungry after 7 p.m. When we sleep at night, the body needs to conduct its internal repairs. If you want to wake up in the morning with clear eyes and head, and ready to face the day, please follow this tip.
9	**EAT** your biggest meal early, preferably around mid-day. Food eaten earlier in the day, when you are more physically active, can be better digested. There's an old saying: "When the sun is highest in the sky, our digestive powers are at their greatest."
10	**CHEW** your food extremely well. Slow and thorough chewing brings forth a greater supply of mouth and digestive enzymes. These catalytic enzymes help predigest food, thereby keeping fatty wastes from being unnecessarily deposited in your cells. Complete and thorough chewing is also needed to finely pulverize food, allowing for better absorption of nutrients and far less effort for the body to digest.
11	**DRINK** juice immediately after preparation. Enzymes begin to evaporate in as little as five minutes. It's called oxidation. So drink your juice as quickly after juicing as possible. If you want to drink your juices away from home, use a stainless steel lined thermos, rinse the inside with water, and pour the water out. Place in the freezer overnight. Make your juice in the morning and take your thermos out of the freezer. You will notice the inside looks frosted. Pour your juice inside and screw on the top. The frozen liner will keep your juice enzyme-rich and stabilized for approximately four to six hours, or until the inside thaws out.
12	**WHEN** drinking digestive juice aids with a cooked meal, always "chew" the first few mouthfuls by swishing it around until it begins to taste sweet. This process helps the salivary glands and taste buds to secrete ptyalin. Ptyalin is an amylase, similar to an enzyme, that will readily initiate the breakdown of carbohydrates into simple sugars and starches, thereby ensuring you extract the full nutritional value of your meal. There is an old doctor friend of mine from the 1940s who used to tell us, "Chew your foods extremely well, at least fifty times per mouthful." This was known as the "Fletcherizer Method." Since we are recommending the digestive juice aids be consumed when you are eating a cooked meal, this chewing can be lessened by at least 70 percent.

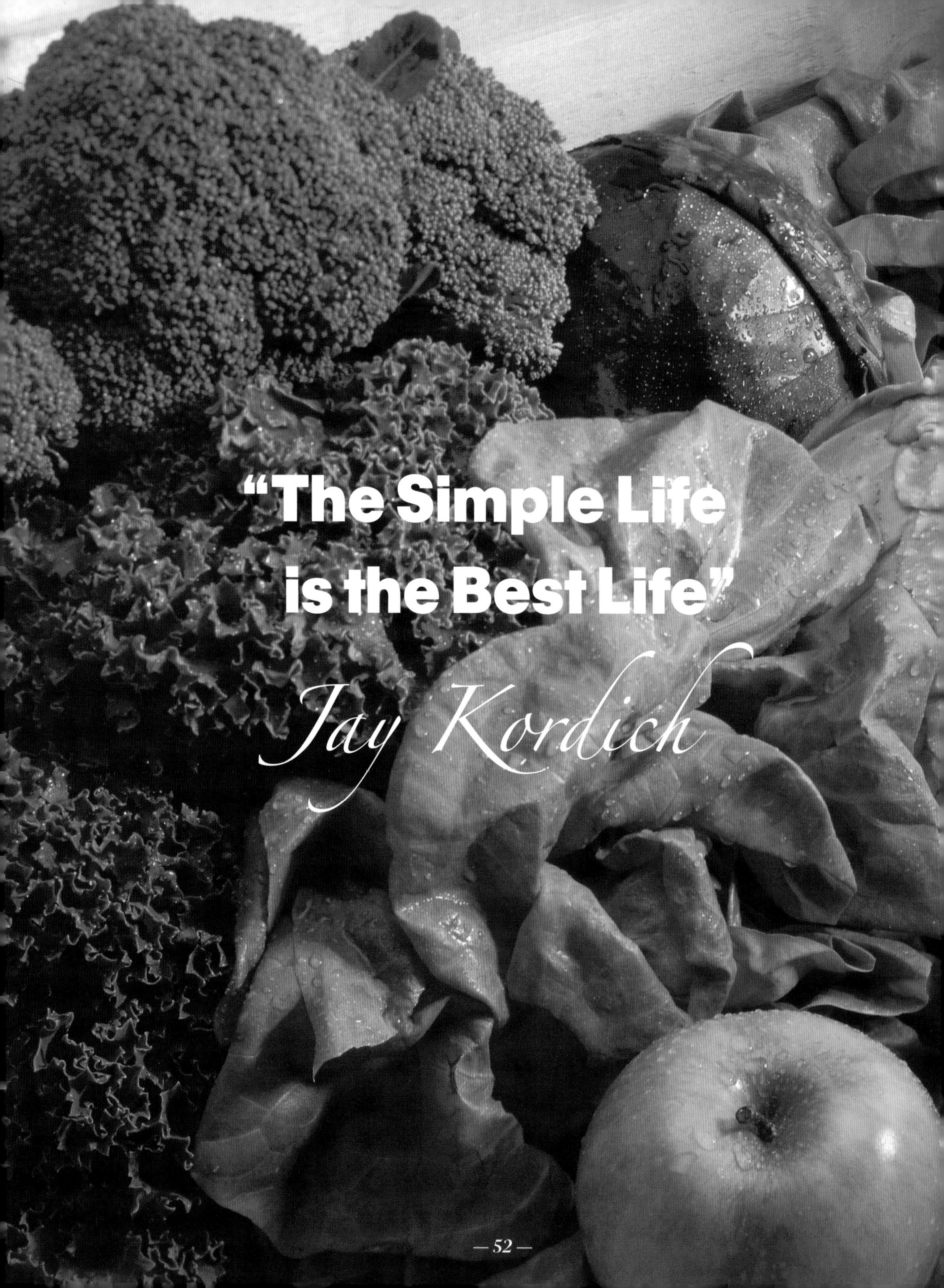

"The Simple Life is the Best Life"

Jay Kordich

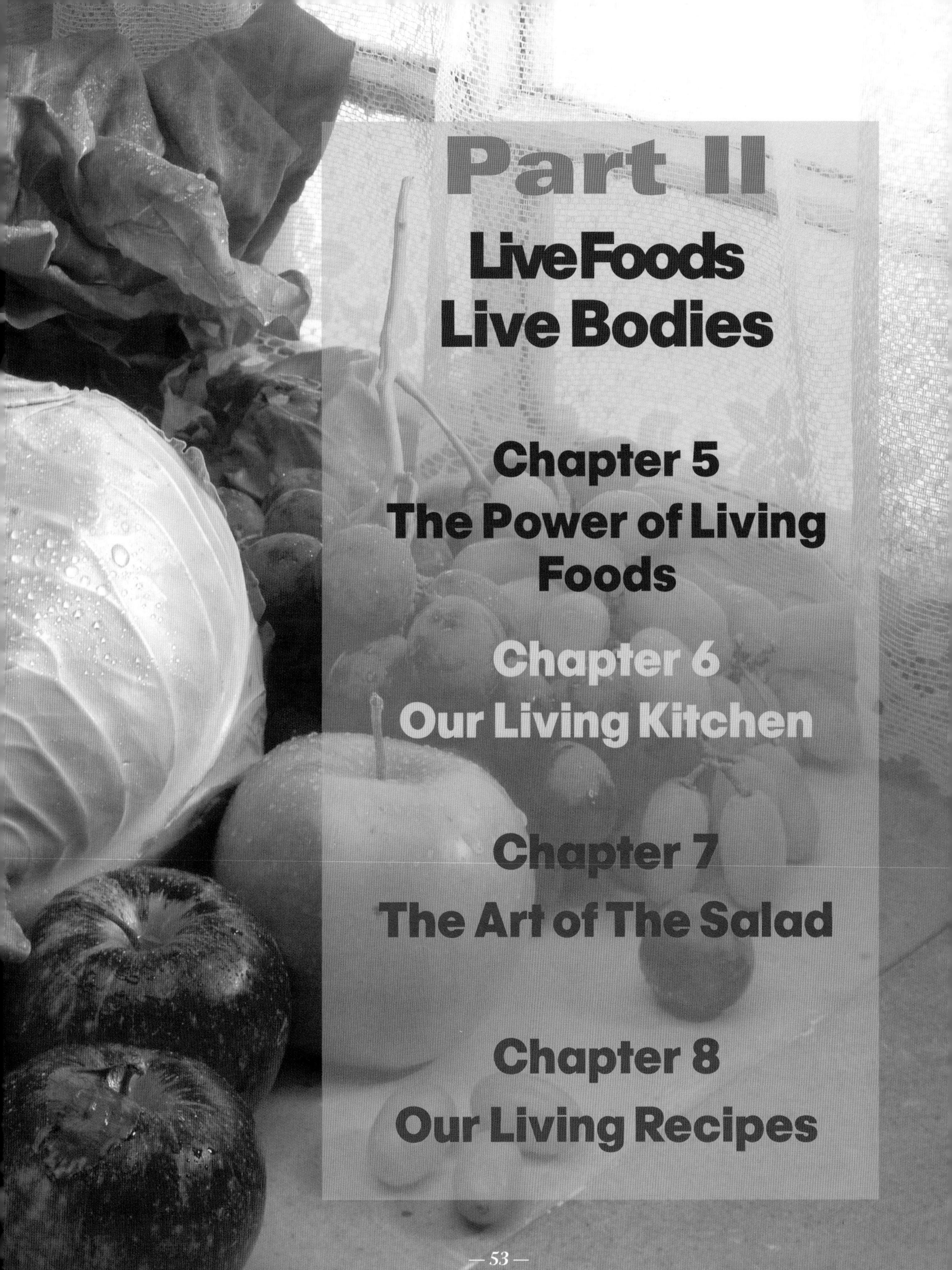

Part II

Live Foods Live Bodies

Chapter 5
The Power of Living Foods

Chapter 6
Our Living Kitchen

Chapter 7
The Art of The Salad

Chapter 8
Our Living Recipes

“We Make Foo

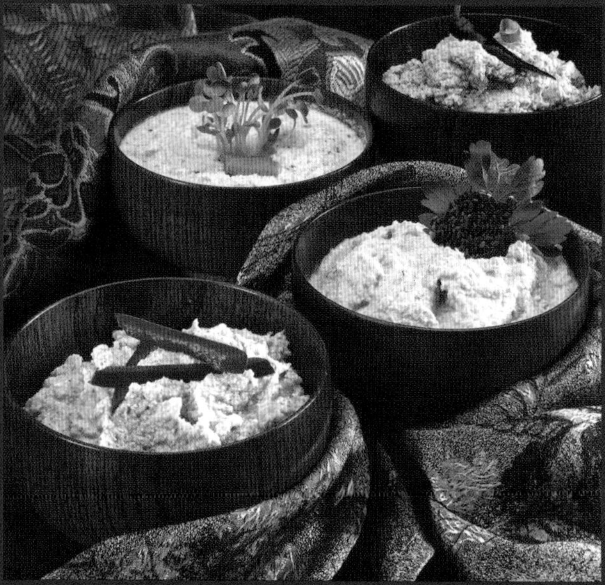

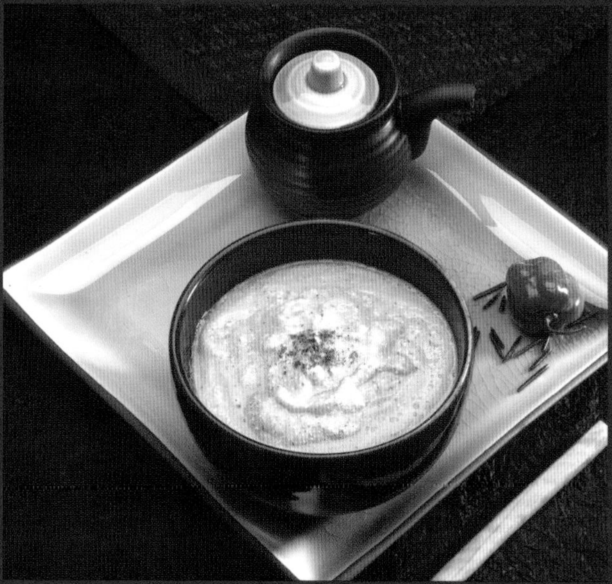

Come Alive!"

Jay Kordich

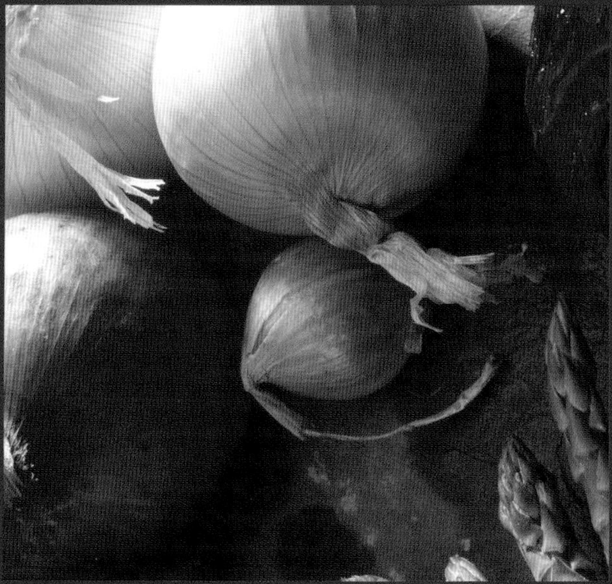

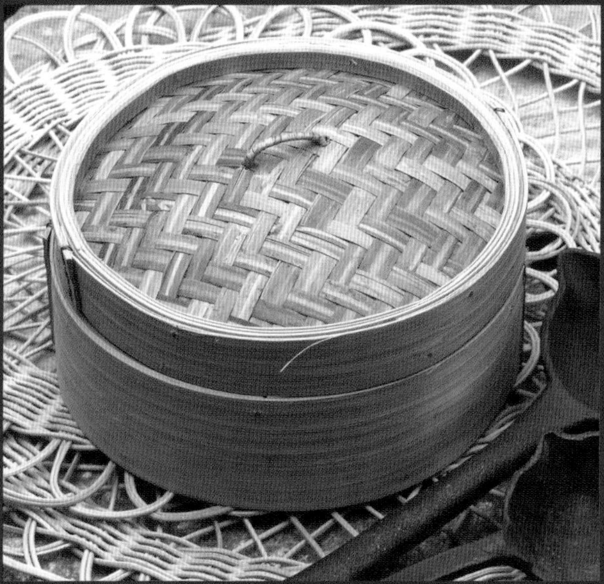

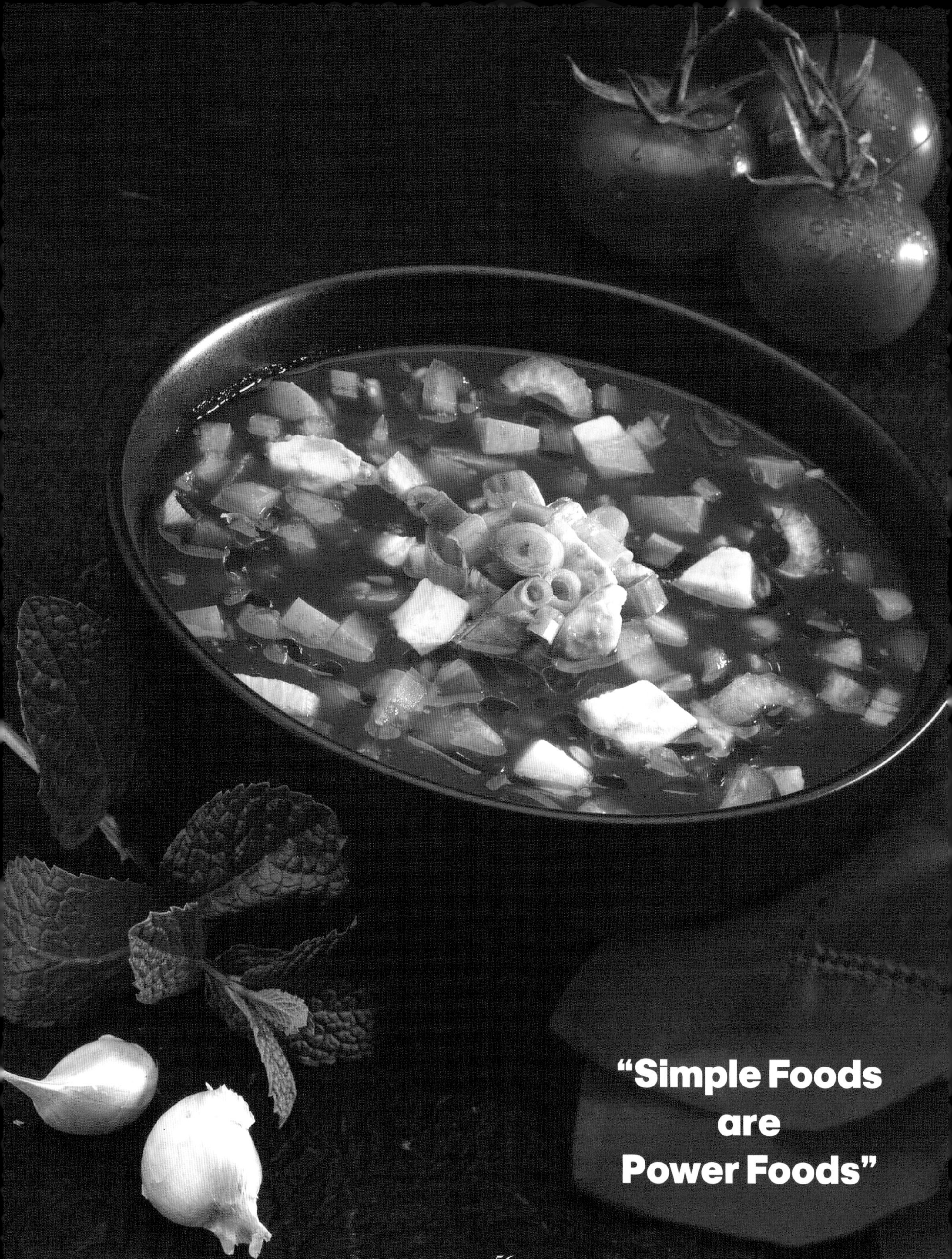
"Simple Foods
are
Power Foods"

Chapter 5
The Power of Living Foods

What *Are* Living Foods?

- The 75/25 Principle
- Acceptable Cooked Foods on Our Program
- Foods, Herbs, and Spices Needed for The Program
- The Importance of Superior Quality Nuts and Oils

That's Me, Linda!

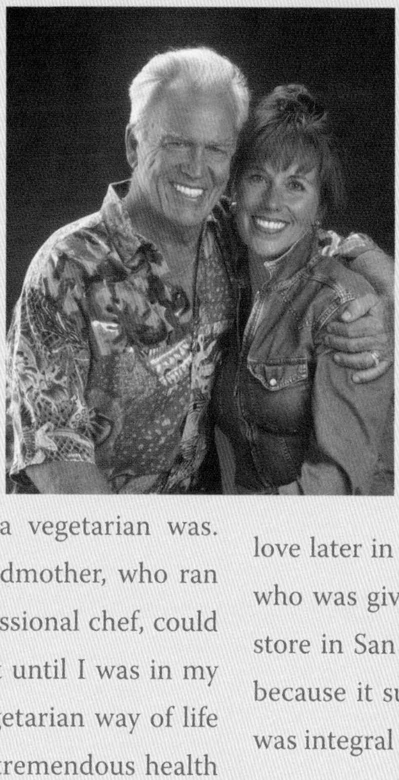

Jay's domain has always been juicing, whereas I have been inspired by the preparation of great-tasting vegetarian food. In 1965, I woke up one day, at the tender age of ten, hearing my mother proudly announce to the family, "We are all going to be vegetarians!"

It didn't really matter to me because I didn't know what a vegetarian was. Besides, I wasn't worried. My grandmother, who ran our household and was also a professional chef, could make anything taste good. It wasn't until I was in my teens that I realized choosing a vegetarian way of life was virtuous, and brought with it, tremendous health advantages.

For me, it's been a dedicated, lifelong choice, but it doesn't mean Jay and I insist you must be a vegetarian. Ultimately, it is a better choice if we want to live more disease-free lifestyles when we reach our fifties throughout the rest of our lives. Research has proven that the longest living cultures such as the Okinawans and the Hunzas eat a predominately vegetarian diet.

By the time I was ten, back in 1965, my mother discovered the powers that lie in fresh vegetable juicing, which intensified our existing healthy eating style. I can remember coming home from junior high school, racing up the front steps and hearing the juicer whirring. At that age, I wasn't exactly fond of drinking vegetable juices, but my mother was smart enough to know she was helping me build a taste for something I would come to absolutely love later in life. By 1978, my mother met Jay Kordich, who was giving a seminar on juicing at a health food store in San Diego. She loved listening to his lectures because it supported her long-held belief that juicing was integral to longevity and vital health.

I Finally Meet Jay

A few years later, I finally met the man my mother had been always talking about – Jay Kordich. He had not been married for close to forty years, and was 32 years older than me. I remember he had the most beautiful skin and physique. Little did I know that on that innocent day in September of 1980, my life would soon change forever.

Several months after I met Jay, I decided I wanted to talk to him about possibly working with him but something strange happened. Somewhere along the conversation we took a left turn. Instead of talking about working together, we started to talk about how we were meant to *be* together. To make a long story short, we got married the next day.

Now, not only was I going to work with Jay, I was also going to be his wife! Strange. I had been somewhat down to earth in life, not venturing out by making wild decisions, but this was destiny. I knew he was going to be my husband, and we were indeed going to have children, and we would travel the United States teaching as many people as possible the wonderful benefits of juice therapy combined with vegetarian eating. However, much to the chagrin of my friends and family back in San Diego, we eloped and traveled the first four years of our marriage, selling juicers and teaching vegetarian food classes all over America. Thus, we began our lifelong mission together teaching our sincere passion for vital health. We had so much fun during those early days.

With my strong background and knowledge in the preparation of vegetarian foods, and with Jay being "The Father of Juicing," it was only natural for the kitchen to

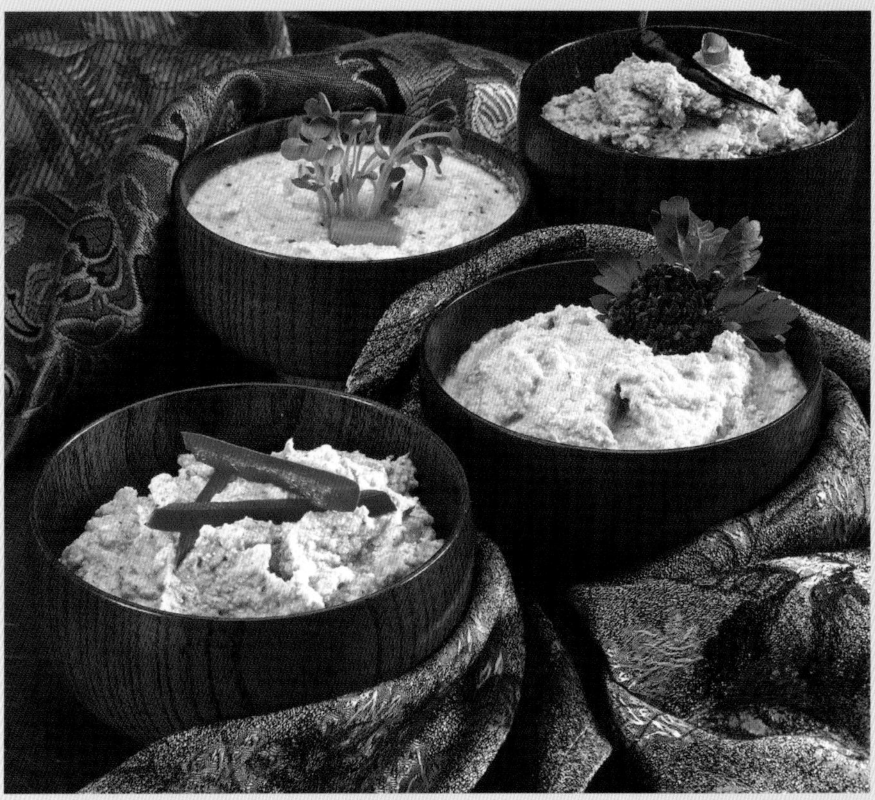

become the center of our universe. While I have a more feminine approach to foods, Jay's attitude is more masculine. We've come to realize our combined approach to food is powerful. Our program allows us to share this wonderful knowledge with others. I like to say that first Jay Kordich brought The Power of Juicing to the world, and now he brings us the Power of Living Foods.

What Jay and I have learned over the years is that eating primarily living foods is crucially important to our vital health, stamina, endurance, and youthful energy. While we are convinced that eating a diet rich in mostly raw, living foods is the best way to live, we are not advocating eating only raw foods.

100% Living is Not Recommended for Beginners

For most people, it's just not a sustainable eating pattern for life. Unless you live in a very warm climate, and your job and lifestyle do not induce stress or strife, the purity of these living foods is not likely to balance nicely with the rest of your life. Mirroring your lifestyle with your food style is the key.

In other words, if you live a stressful life and drink coffee and alcohol regularly, then a diet of 100 percent living foods may not work for you. But incorporating a larger percentage of living foods into your diet is the attainable goal of our program, and that's how we live. If I have been under stress or gained a few unwanted pounds, sometimes I will go on two or three week diet of 100 percent living foods. But we have found that as we pass through different seasons, our bodies requires some cool foods and some hot foods, so we have designed our 75/25 program to fit for life, rather than for a few weeks. In chapter 3, you will be able to take our test to see what type of transition diet will work best for you, and how easy it will be for you to make the transition into a greener diet.

Adopting a living food lifestyle can also be a jump start for change in different aspects of our life, unrelated to food choices. You may find that when we make small adjustments to our food choices, our inner senses begin to see and hear differently. Our taste buds start to change. We become attracted to nature on a more regular basis. We start to crave greens and vegetable juices. We become calmer in our demeanors. These are the things that naturally change within us, and each of us is different. For some, it's an immediate change. For others, it may take about two weeks to a month.

As you will discover in the chapters ahead, our bodies crave emotional nourishment as well as physical nourishment. In chapter 7 I painfully share the trauma I endured during my high school and college days, suffering from an eating disorder. This is why I know so much about emotional healing through foods and about how addicted we can become to foods, sometimes without even being aware of it. It's not just what we eat, it's also what kind of relationship we have with ourselves and the foods we eat. I can joyfully say I've been free from this addiction for twenty two years.

What Are Living Foods?

Before we launch into the program, let's discuss the most important issue: What *are* living foods?

Living foods are plant foods such as nuts, seeds, grains, herbs, fruits, and vegetables, including greens, eaten or juiced in their natural form without cooking. Mother Nature sun bakes our plant food to perfection, so it is best to consume these foods with their naturally intrinsic values intact. In this way, all the life-giving vitamins, minerals, and enzymes inherent in them can be absorbed.

When food is cooked above 119 degrees Fahrenheit, all enzymes are killed, which critically degrades the food's vitality, ultimately arresting good digestion and depleting our natural supplies of our own enzyme bank accounts. Unfortunately, most ovens

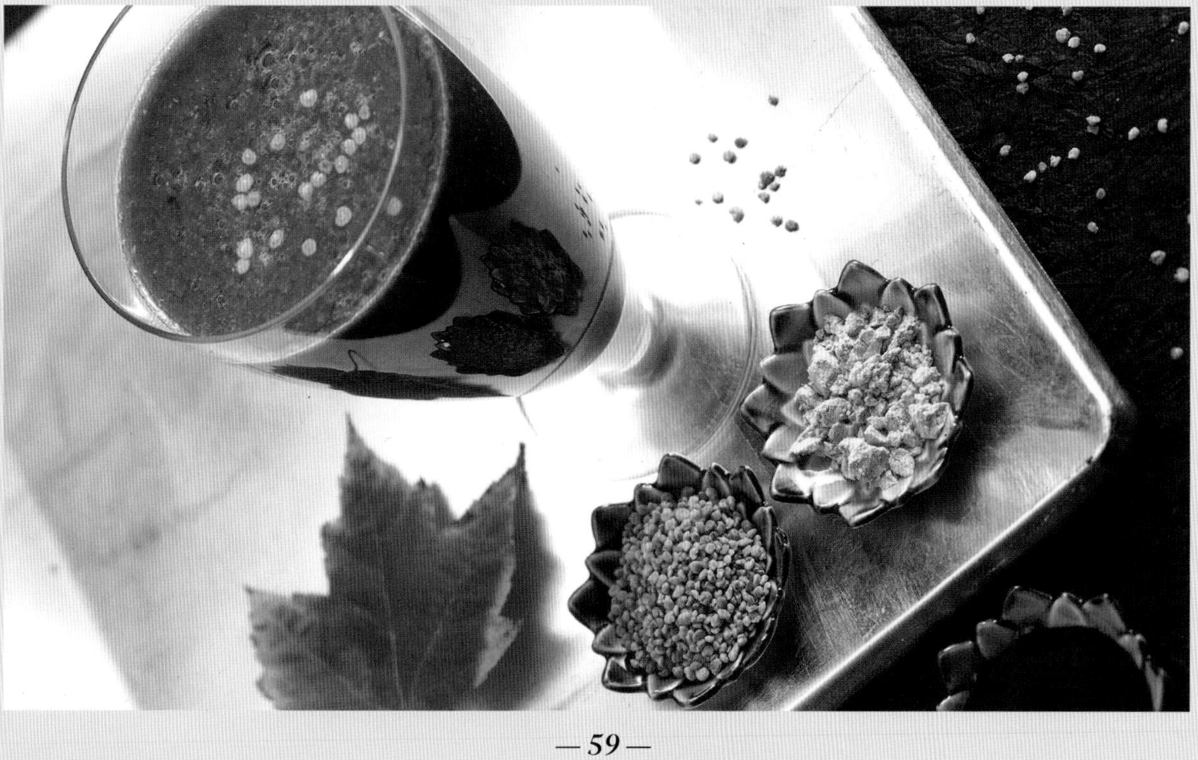

begin at 220 degrees Fahrenheit, thereby eliminating the need for the conventional ovens. However, we love our dehydrator, which will never go over 115 degrees, and we mention on page 82.

While some foods are perfect just off the vine, other foods like broccoli, cauliflower, and green beans can benefit from a bit of steaming. This makes them easier to chew and removes some of the hidden fungus that could be present. A bit of steaming means to cook for only one or two minutes after the water comes to a boil in the steamer. The vegetables become crisp-tender and retain their bright color.

Later in this chapter, we will identify which foods require special preparation. You will be surprised to see how effortlessly these small changes can be accomplished.

Why Would You Want to Follow a Living Foods/Raw Diet?

One of the best reasons for you to try a living foods/raw diet is the exhilaration you can feel with how much vital energy awaits you, and it starts to happen within 48 hours. Your stamina may increase, and your bowel habits may change dramatically in a very positive, "regular" way. What's more, your skin may start to improve, and natural weight loss occurs for most people. But most rewarding is the development of a natural calmness in your demeanor. A relaxed attitude starts to lighten your spirits, and addictions to foods such as sugar, caffeine, wheat products, and processed foods start to disappear! Is that great, or what?

On a more serious note, imagine how many animals will not have to suffer a horrible death due to your dietary choices, and imagine how beautiful you will feel inside and out when you begin having all these wonderful experiences. You will actually start living in harmony with nature, and yourself. This is the legacy awaiting you. Within two to three weeks on this program, you will start to notice big changes, and within three months, you can overcome all addictions to poor food habits. You could be on your way to increased vital health, stamina, and true balanced energy for as long as you wish. Isn't it worth a try? Just remember, if you go back to eating sugar, caffeine or white flour products, it unfortunately triggers our old food addictions, thereby setting us on a negative and frustrating road. But the good news is that if this happens, (and it does for a lot of us) you now know how to de-activate the addictions by just getting back on your living foods program.

Our 75/25 Principle

Cooked foods digest better when combined with up to 75 percent living foods. This means that in the fall and winter, 75 percent of our meals are prepared with living foods, and 25 percent are cooked. This is what we call the 75/25 Principle. In the spring and summer, we tend to eat more toward an 80 percent living foods meal, while 20 percent of our meal is cooked.

When we refer to either 25 percent or 20 percent cooked foods, we don't mean lunch meat or cookies! Our acceptable cooked foods are mostly (soaked) cooked grains and legumes, lightly steamed vegetables, cooked soups, and tofu. Sometimes during the winter months, we consume more warming foods because the weather calls for it. On pages 5 in this chapter, you will see our acceptable cooked foods chart.

Eating according to the seasons is very important to Jay and me. Seasons have a way of telling us what to eat, naturally. For example, in October, when pears, pomegranates, and squashes are in season, we automatically know that we should be eating more of them. Likewise, during the summer months, we'll consume perfectly ripe foods like peaches, cherries, berries, green beans, and tomatoes.

We Need to Build a Good Relationship with Natural Foods

Part of our dysfunction towards empowering us with good eating habits is the fact, pure, and simple, most of us do *NOT* have a good relationship with natural foods. We don't know all the varieties of fruits and vegetables that await us. Truthfully, we are not to blame. Most of us didn't have mothers who were home teaching us these wonderful skills, and we ourselves don't seem to have time, or do we? Think about it for a minute. All we need to do is prioritize our time just a bit.

When I started to learn the secrets of natural foods, I started to realize Mother Nature shares a beautiful experience through four seasons every year, showering us with her different rainbow colored varieties of fruits and vegetables. When our food habits start to flow with the seasons, we start to connect to nature in ways we would not have imagined. Our senses about life start to change. We become more aware of quiet and hidden ambiances we may never have noticed, like wind flowing gently and lovingly through our hair. Birds begin to romance us with their songs if we closely listen. Once we start to flow with the seasons, and start to eat more natural foods, our bodies will respond and feel more alive. It can become a beautiful experience when we start to balance our lives with nature. It may sound corny, but once you experience this, your attitude about these things will start to change. However, if we are busy being distracted by choosing to eat in fast food restaurants, making poor food choices in supermarkets, stressing ourselves out trying to figure out how to get unstressed, we miss these wonderful, free and liberating experiences awaiting us.

Even the Experts Agree

Understanding why living foods are so important takes time. It requires "unlearning" what we've blindly deemed acceptable for many years. However, most people—even in the medical profession—will attest to the fact that the less we cook our foods, the more nutrients, vitamins, minerals, and especially enzymes are preserved.

Jay and I have undergone many years of evolution to arrive at the living foods health-style we've come to value. We recognize that changing our eating habits is a very personal journey. By sharing with you what we know to be true about living foods and why they are so important to your vital health, we hope to shorten your evolution toward more enlightening food choices. After all, we have been studying and living this lifestyle for close to 90 combined years. In chapter 6, when you start our Living Kitchen program, you'll appreciate this endearing yet powerful way of living. Sometimes we change for the better, and then sometimes we regress a bit. What's important is consistently coming back to these healthier eating habits. The more you do, the better you become are at getting closer and closer to your ultimate goal-a well balanced life.

Your Own Personal Journey Can Begin Now

After you finish this program, you will begin to start your own personal journey to becoming a master of your own food habits and skills. (See back of recipe section-pages just for you.) Don't be too hard on yourself if you slip up every now and then. Jay had an easy transition to eating fresh fruits and vegetables, as the urgent threat of cancer compelled him to serious commitment and attention. I took longer—about three years—because I came from a strong vegetarian household where a cooked food, vegetarian way of eating prevailed.

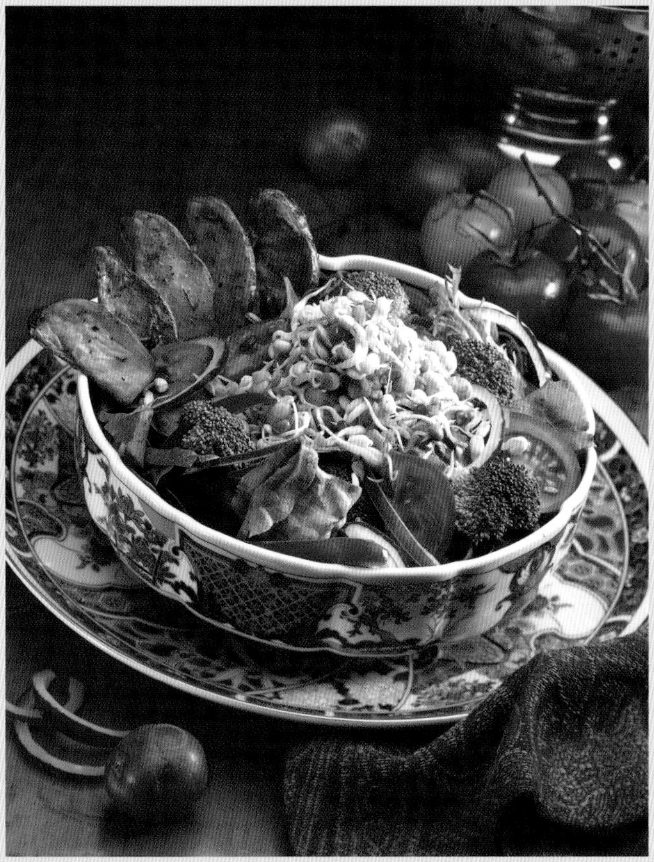

Our 75%/25% Living Foods Program

Our 75/25 cooked transition diet is achieved by adding any of the following cooked grains with any fresh, raw salad. If you eat more than 50% of your food 'living' the cooked foods digest better. We suggest mixing the grains right into the salad. You'll be tickled at how delicious and satisfying a salad-eating experience can be with the simple addition of a cooked grain, or even nuts, seeds, or cooked beans. On page 95 you will see Jay and I have designed a Super Salad Pyramid, displaying all the examples of foods you can add to turn your regular, boring salad into a Super Salad, or Whole Meal Salad, however you like to see it. I like to call them Super Salads because they are bigger than life to some people who come to our house and taste them. I can tell they have never eaten a meal such as ours. Next listed is our list of acceptable cooked grains to add to your living foods program: We do not recommend white rice of any kind. White rice has been stripped of all its nutritive values, then the manufacturers add in synthetic vitamins and minerals. Best to stay with the complex carbohydrates in our grains, rather than the simple carbohydrates such as white rice. The only foods we eat that are white in color are potatoes and tofu. And with potatoes, the only way we eat them, considering they are a simple carbohydrate, is combined in salads. Tofu is not considered a simple carbohydrate.

25% Acceptable Cooked Grains

- Brown rice (short and long grain)
- Bulghur (cracked wheat from mid east))
- Millet (small grained cereal))
- Pearl barley (pearlized barley grain)
- Quinoa (ancient grain from the Andes))
- Oats (groats, steel cut and regular)
- Buckwheat noodles and/or Cous Cous

Keeping these grains on hand supports your ability to create an entire meal within minutes. It's wise to rinse thoroughly and soak these grains in steamed distilled/purified water the night before or at least two hours before cooking. However, cut oats only need fifteen minutes or so. (We only use cut oats in breakfasts such as muesli, and not in salads.) Soaking is very important because it releases an enzyme inhibitor, which then allows for much better absorption and digestion. You can prepare one of the above grains as you get ready for work or the night before.

Try purchasing an automatic rice maker with which you can make various types of grains, including brown rice. It's easier to prepare your grains the night before with one of these appliances. Make sure to purchase only high quality appliances. Cheaper models will contain an aluminum body. Jay and I are very wary of purchasing any product containing aluminum, even inside rice cookers. They are hard to find but worth the effort. (Panasonic or Zojirushi are brand names worth looking into.) By the time you come home from work, you will only have to prepare the salad.

The magic of a satisfying salad is accomplished by varying the different dressings and cooked grains, nuts, seeds, sprouts, steamed veggies and tofu, combined with the green salad ingredients. It may sound confusing as you read this, but within time you will see just how easy it is to teach yourself how to make wholemeal salads.

You'll find it easy to get started with our recipes in chapter 8 and our Salad Pyramid is beautifully displayed for easy understanding. As you become more proficient in salad preparation, you'll find it exciting to explore new combinations on your own! The most important point to remember is not to put your salad dressings onto the Super Salad until you are prepared to eat it. Our children sometimes like to wrap the entire meal up in a tortilla (warmed up) then put the dressing over the salad, then wrap it up into a burrito shaped meal. This is recommended for teenagers or children above the age of three years old. Children and teenagers enjoy eating their salads this way, and frankly it's a great way to get them started on a high fiber diet. Try purchasing colored tortillas to make it more joyful, but be very careful to read the ingredients, as most colored tortillas actually have unnatural red dyes' or blue dye's, which to us is shocking, but there is not a law that prohibits food manufacturers from doing this. We need to be aware and always read labels on all the foods we purchase that are packaged. There is research that shows artificial colors and artificial preservatives wreck havoc in the nervous systems of children, causing all kinds of behavioral disorders, including adults too.

As we listen, read and analyze, we evolve by making better food choices, and so does the rest of the world. Remember on page 103 we spoke about using the media in ways that helps humanity? This is how we change, the world for our children and their children's children. *We* have the power, to make foods more pure, organic and safe.

Tips for Great Cooked Soups

- ***To** make a soup seem richer, add a bit of olive oil on the top before serving.*
- ***If** your soup looks too thin, add cooked brown rice or cooked pearl barley as a thickener.*
- ***Don't** use bouillon cubes. Unless they are vegetarian based, they can be rancid and beef or chicken based. If desired, use any of the tasty vegetable-based seasonings made by Gayelord Hauser or Dr. Jensen's seasonings (available at most grocery and health food stores). Follow package directions for making instant vegetable stock.*
- ***Mushrooms** are a great addition to make your soup more "beefy" tasting.*
- ***Dried** herbs are good for most soups.*
- ***Fresh** herbs are best used in soups only as a garnish or stirred in just before serving to preserve their full flavor and goodness.*
- ***Ideally,** wait at least six hours to serve soups so all their flavors can blend.*
- ***When** storing soups, put them either in the freezer or refrigerator. Keep soup in the refrigerator for no more than three days.*
- ***Leftover** homemade soups make great lunches for work, so freeze in individual serving containers for easy thawing and use.*
- ***If** soup is allowed to sit overnight (in the fridge), natural salt flavors from the vegetables steep and prevent over salting.*

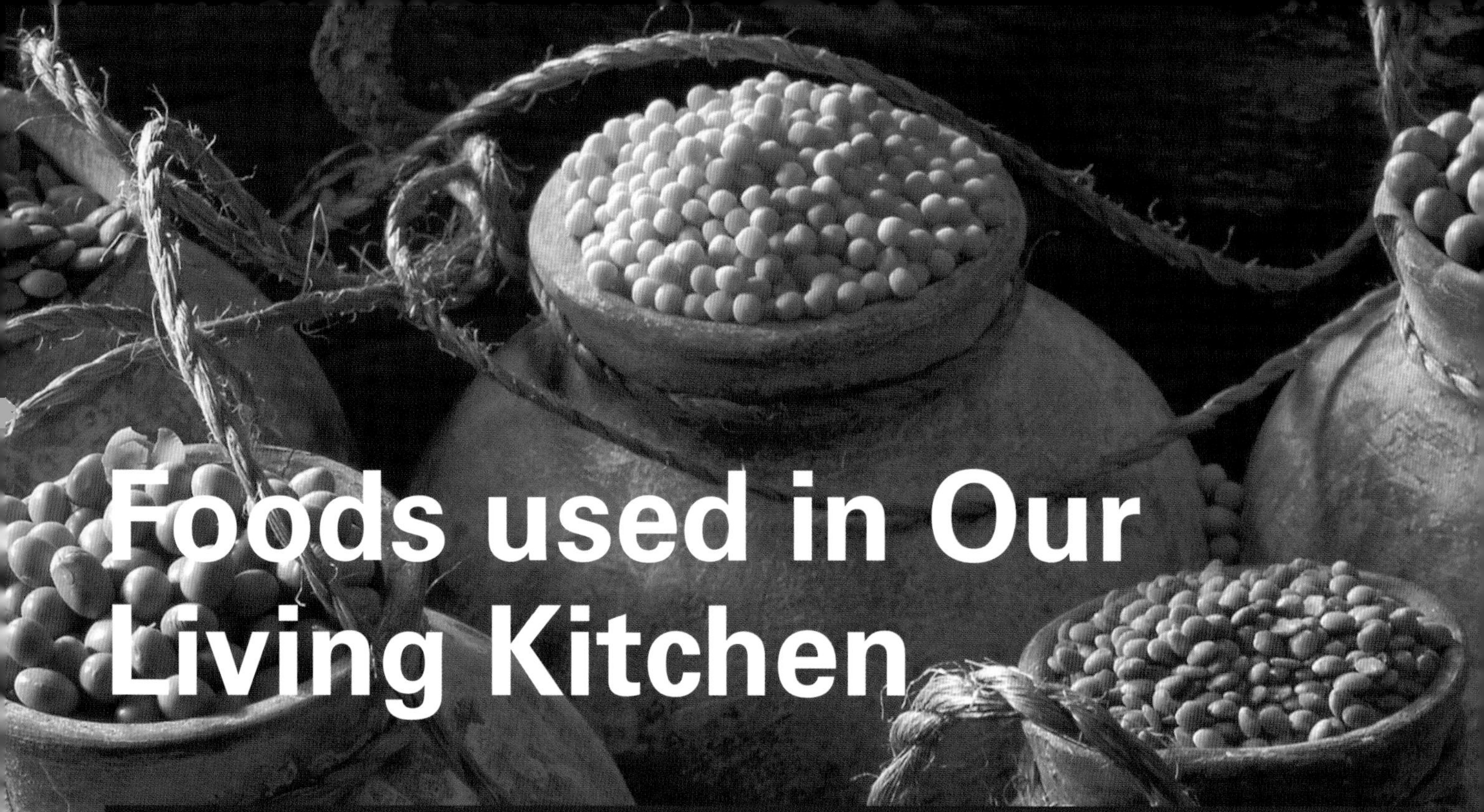

Foods used in Our Living Kitchen

1	Organic Dried or Bottled Spices Used in Our Living Kitchen	• Bay leaves • Black pepper • Cayenne pepper • Celery seed • Cinnamon • Cumin • Curry • Herbs de Province • Nutmeg • Oregano • Paprika • Sage • Sea salt (Celtic is best.) • Organic vanilla extract
2	Organic Fresh Herbs/Roots Used in Our Living Kitchen	• Basil • Chives • Cilantro • Clove • Dill • Fennel • Garlic • Ginger • Marjoram • Oregano • Parsley • Peppermint • Rosemary • Sage • Spearmint • Tarragon • Thyme
3	Fresh Herbal Teas	• Peppermint • Spearmint • Chamomile • Ginger • Green • Echinacea • Dandelion • Eucha-mint • Ginseng
4	Nut Butters	• Walnuts • Almonds • Sunflower seeds • Sesame seeds • Pecans • Flax seeds • Filberts • Pumpkin seeds • Macadamia nuts
5	Grains	• Short grain brown rice • Long grain brown rice • Quinoa • Millet • Kashi • Pearl barley • Bulghur • Oats, steel cut and rolled • CousCous
6	Beans	• Adzuki beans • Garbanzo beans • White navy beans • Pinto beans • Kidney beans • Black eyed peas • Lentils—green, red, and yellow • French lentils • Mung beans • Black beans

7	Sprouts	• Alfalfa • Mung bean • Adzuki • Lentil • Barley • Bean • Garbanzo • Fenugreek • Triticale • Wheat • Sunflower • Broccoli
8	Organic Vegetables Used in Our Living Kitchen	• Asparagus • Alfalfa sprouts • Beets • Beet greens • Bell peppers • Broccoli • Broccoli sprouts • Brussels sprouts • Cabbage (red and green) • Carrots • Cauliflower • Celery • Collard greens • Chard (green Swiss, red, or rainbow) • Cucumbers • Corn • Dandelion greens • Fennel • Ginger • Green beans • Green onions • Garlic • Jalapeno • Jicima • Kale • Leeks • Mixed baby organic greens • Mung bean sprouts • Mushrooms (shitake) • Napa cabbage • Onions • Onion sprouts • Parsley • Peppers: yellow, red, and orange • Anaheim peppers • Peas • Pea shoots, fresh • Potatoes; red, brown, white, and yellow • Pumpkin • Radicchio • Radishes • Romaine lettuce • Spinach • Sprouted legumes (garbanzo, lentil, peas, etc.) • Squashes (butternut, banana, acorn, turban, summer squash • Kombucha (my favorite) • Sunflower seed sprouts • Sweet potatoes • Turnips • Turnip greens • Vine ripened tomatoes: red, yellow, orange • Zucchini, green and yellow
9	Organic Specialty Items for Our Living Kitchen	• Apple cider vinegar (organic) • Balsamic vinegar • Borage and flax seed oils (refrigerated) • Bragg's Liquid Aminos • Capers • Edamame (soy beans in pods) • Essene breads (living breads) • Grape seed oil • Green tea soba noodles • Herbal teas in bulk form • Macadamia nut oil • Maple syrup (organic) • Miso, red, white, and brown • Olive oil (extra virgin) • Pumpkin seed oil • Rice milks (organic) • Soy milks (organic) • Soy sauce (organic, raw, and unpasteurized called nama shoyu) • Sucanant • Sun dried tomatoes • Tamari (wheat free nama shoyu) • Tofu (fresh) soft, firm, and extra firm • Wheat grass (freshly grown)
10	Specialty Fruits, Fresh and Dried	• Young, baby coconuts • Fresh figs • Fresh dates • Olives (organic) Green and Black • Dried fruits (non-sulfites): Apricots, Figs, Cranberries, Raisins, Cherries, Blueberries, Gooseberries

Organic Fruit

Jay and I try to always keep our fruits out on the kitchen counter, except our juicing apples. Apples juice better when cold, but we love to eat Fuji apples and keep them on the counter along with the other fruits. Other exceptions are berries. Berries must be kept cold because they are fragile. Most fruits ripen better at room temperature, which enhances their flavor and fragrance. Some fruits ripen faster than others. If you decide to keep a big bowl of fruit in your kitchen, here are a few suggestions to keep in mind:

1. Fruits naturally ripen because they emit a natural gas called ethylene. Ethylene gas can cause vegetables to age too quickly if in close proximity to fruits.
2. Apples and watermelon are the only fruits that do not emit ethylene gases.
3. We keep bananas separate on a banana hanger. This helps them ripen on their own and without getting bruised.

We recommend that you read the following list to make sure these are the fruits you keep on your counter top and away from apples, watermelon, and most vegetables. (We refrigerate our apples.

· Apricots · Avocados · Bananas · Cantaloupes · Casaba melons · Grapes green, red, concord) · Honeydew melons · Kiwis · Mangoes · Nectarines · Papayas · Peaches · Pears · Plums · Tomatoes

Just remember not to put your veggies and fruits together, either in a bowl on the table or together in the refrigerator. (Tomatoes and avocados are considered fruits.)

Fruits Used in Our Living Kitchen

· Apples
· Apricots
· Bananas, red and yellow
· Blackberries
· Blueberries
· Cantaloupes
· Casaba melons
· Cherries
· Coconuts, baby and regular
· Cranberries
· Dried fruits (apricots, cherries, figs, raisins, etc.),
· Fresh figs
· Grapes (red, green, concord)
· Grapefruits
· Honeydews
· Kiwis
· Lemons
· Limes
· Mangos
· Nectarines
· Oranges
· Papayas
· Peaches
· Pears
· Pineapple
· Plums
· Pomegranates
· Raspberries
· Star fruits
· Strawberries
· Tangelos
· Tangerines
· Watermelons

Vegetarian Eating Styles

Should you like to explore a specific vegetarian eating style, there are different kinds of vegetarian eating regimes. If you already are a vegetarian, you may be interested in trying a different style of vegetarianism. Listed here are various vegetarian eating styles and the types of foods eaten within those styles. But first, here are a few points you should know:

We would like to caution parents of children committed to vegetarian lifestyles that it is not desirable if their children are choosing to eat doughnuts and Twinkies just because they're not animals. Kids need good protein foods, such as tofu, soybeans, sprouted grains, soaked nuts, greens in many different forms (especially in juice form), salads, fresh fruits, and steamed distilled water—every day. This goes for adults also, but it is especially important for teenagers. Teenagers have a tendency to skip meals and make unwise food choices. This can lead to an unbalanced vegetarian diet. If you want to support them in their new eating habits, we suggest they do some research to see what an appropriate vegetarian eating lifestyle looks like. They can either go to our site, jaykordich.com or to the Google search engine and pull up vegetarian foods. You will find countless web sites and articles on vegetarian foods

1. Fruitarian:

Consumes only fruits, nuts, seeds, and berries. Sometimes they consume cooked grains. Fruitarians eat only plant foods that are harvested from the plant without killing it.

2. 100% Living Foodist/Vegan

Consumes only uncooked nuts, seeds, fruits, vegetables, herbs, and some sprouted legumes.

3. 100% Living Foods with Dairy

Same foods as fruitarian, but they would add all dairy products that are unpasteurized.

4. 75/25% Living Foodist

75-80 percent of foods living. Same as 100 percent living foodist-20-25 percent cooked grains and vegetables, including or excluding dairy .

5. Vegan:

100 percent cooked or living foods (plant based) nuts, seeds, fruits, vegetables, grains, legumes, and herbs. No honey, dairy products, or foods derived from or containing animal flesh/ products. Some vegans also refrain from using leather products of any kind

6. Vegetarian:

100 percent cooked or living foods, nuts, seeds, fruits, vegetables, grains, legumes, herbs, dairy, and eggs. No foods derived from or containing animal flesh/products.

7. Lacto Vegetarian:

100 percent vegetarian diet. Consumes any kind of dairy products, but no eggs. (Eggs are not dairy products. They are unborn chickens).

8. Lacto-Ovo Vegetarian:

100 percent vegetarian, but consume all dairy products, including eggs.

9. Pescetarian:

Consume 100 percent vegetarian foods, but consider fish as the only animal source. May consume dairy products.

10. Semi-Vegetarian:

Consume 100 percent vegetarian foods, eggs, fish, fowl, only uncooked nuts, seeds, fruits, vegetables, herbs and some sprouted legumes. No red meats or any other land animal.

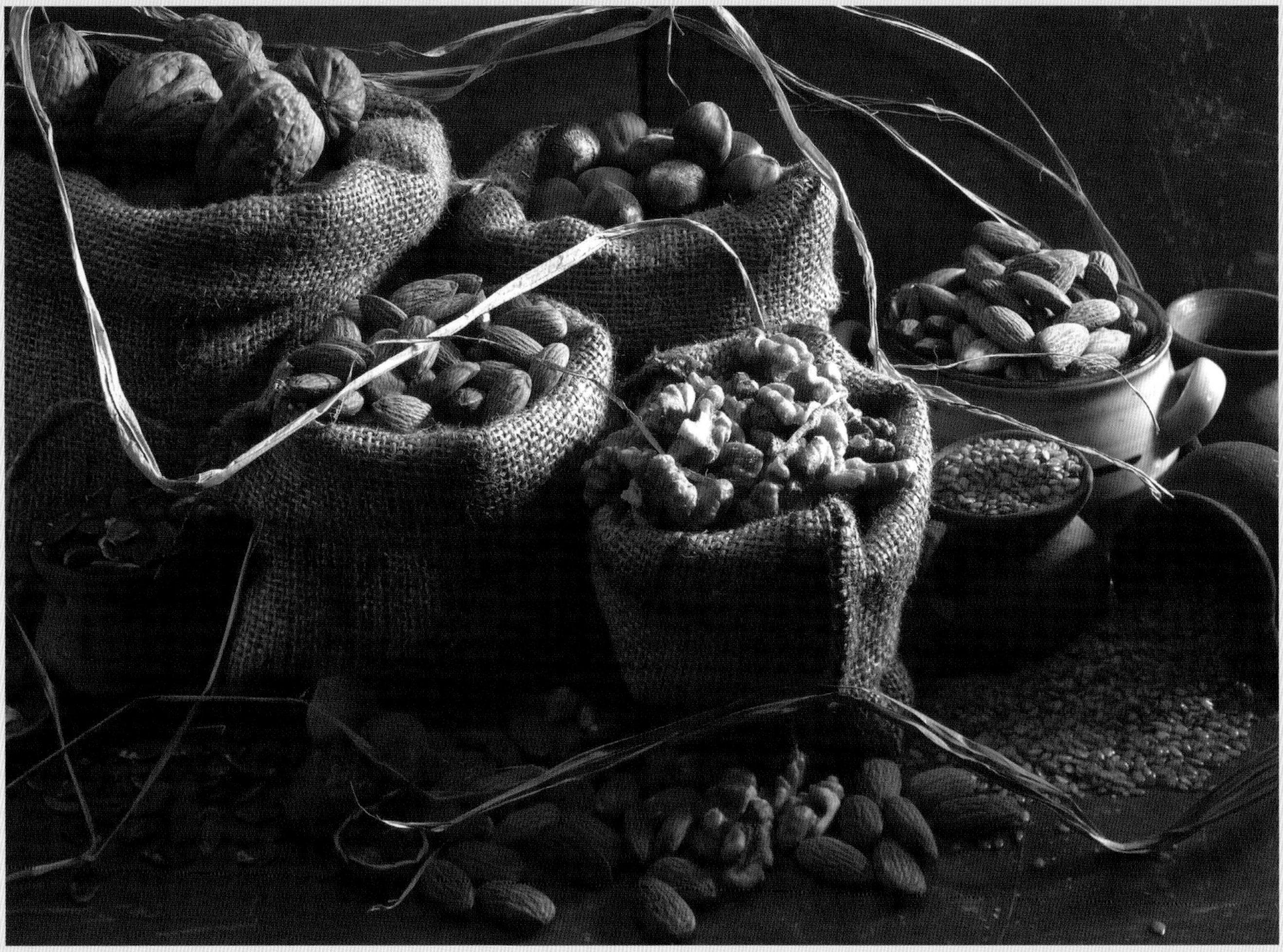

All about Nuts

For many years, it's been reported that nuts should be rarely eaten because of their high fat and calorie content. Few knew the true health benefits and longevity factors that lay inside these wonderful foods. The proven advantages include helping to prevent heart disease and diabetes. Jay and I have always eaten a wide variety of nuts, including almonds, walnuts, pine nuts, pecans, filberts, Brazil nuts, cashews, macadamia nuts, and baby coconuts.

It is best to refrigerate all of your nuts. They stay fresher and will not go rancid or become infested by bugs. In fact, try to purchase your nuts already refrigerated. If this is not possible, be sure to purchase nuts already in packages. Buying in bulk form only risks bringing the bugs home.

More good news about nuts comes from the Harvard School of Public Health researchers, who studied more than 83,000 women. They found that those who ate nuts or peanut butter fives times per week or more, significantly lowered their risk for type 2 diabetes compared with those who never or rarely consumed nuts or peanut butter. (Peanuts are not considered nuts; they are considered legumes.) The women who reported eating nuts at least five times a week reduced their risk by almost 30 percent, and women who frequently ate peanut butter reduced their risk by almost 20 percent. (Journal of the American Medical Associations, 2002, vol. 288, no 20). Just remember, as we said before peanuts are a legume, however we do eat peanut butter in our live foods/live bodies program, but only in its raw form. For example: peanuts are mostly roasted. We do not recommend roasting nuts, ever. And please, never purchase peanut butter with ingredients such as: (hydrogenated oils added). Eating foods and oils with these oils are extremely dangerous to our health.

Fats in nuts are "good," or mono- and

polyunsaturated fats. If you are concerned that they are calorie-dense, be assured that if you add just a handful to salads or cooked grains, or just munch them with your meal, nuts can play an important, satisfying role in your diet. They make a wonderful cheese or meat substitute. In fact, Jay and I use nut pâtés made out of several nuts. You will find our wonderful nut pâté recipes in chapter 8.

Just as it is essential to soak grains and beans for optimal digestion, nuts and seeds are best soaked overnight in steamed distilled water to release natural enzyme inhibitors and promote premium assimilation. If nuts, seeds, and nut/seed butters are eaten raw and unsoaked, digestive enzymes are required to aid digestion so as not to deplete the body's precious metabolic enzyme reserve, making us feel sleepy.

Once nuts and seeds are soaked, pour off the water, rinse, and store in a covered glass container in the fridge. They generally keep for 2-3 days, so it's best to soak the amount you will consume in that time.

Oils—A Very Important Message

One of the most important health changes you can make to your life is to look in your kitchen and see what kind of cooking oils you are using. Only recently has there been attention paid to how harmful hydrogenated oils are, but equally important is the way commonly used oils are processed.

Oils are highly sensitive to processing. In their natural state, oils are rich in proteins and contain highly beneficial Omega 3 and Omega 6 fatty acids, which stimulate the formation of prostaglandins that, in turn, control reproduction, inflammation, immunity, and community between cells, and they prevent over clotting of blood. But their benefits can be negatively affected by extraction methods that employ heat and refinement. Clear bottling can allow light to affect quality and freshness.

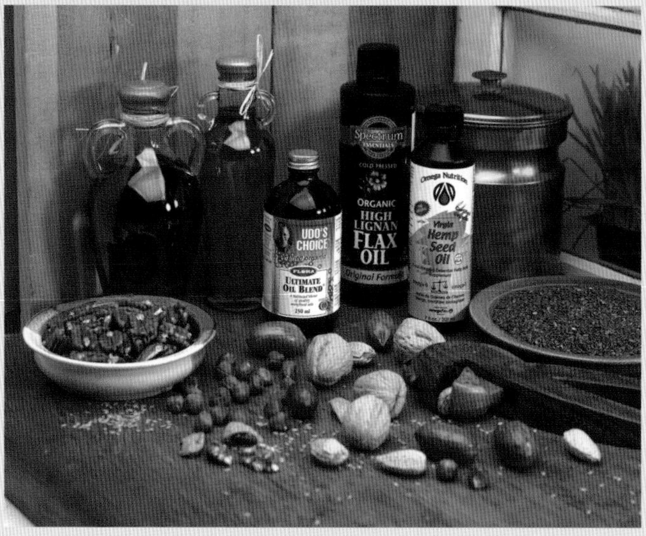

Unrefined oils that are expeller or mechanically pressed and cold-pressed oils go through the least processing and are the most natural, since no heat is used in production. Only about half to three quarters of the oil in a seed or nut can be extracted using the mechanical action of an expeller press to "cold press" the seeds or nuts. These oils are typically more expensive because less oil is obtained using this process. Heating the seeds or nuts until they are slightly roasted yields more oil, as does the solvent extracting method, whereby chemicals draw out almost all oil from the seed or nut. But non-heat produced oils are healthier because they retain more of the inherent nutrients and flavor in the oil.

Solvent extracted oil is a second pressing from the first pressing residue. Even though a petroleum chemical is used and is almost completely burned off in processing, this is surprisingly still considered an unrefined oil. Solvent extracted oils use chemicals that can draw out almost all oil from a seed or nut. Refined oils offer the worst nutritive value since they are produced using high temperatures and synthetic preservatives, and must undergo so many bleaching and chemical solvent processes that they result in a clear, odorless oil almost totally devoid of nutrients. The carcinogenic chemical preservatives are present in small quantities, so their disclosure on the label is not required.

Another point to consider when choosing oils is the temperature at which the oil starts to smoke when heated. When an oil reaches its smoke point, it immediately turns into a trans-fatty oil with the assurability of damaging our heart and arteries. Moreover, heating cooking oils to their smoke point can cause serious indoor air pollution. The lower the smoke point of an oil, the quicker that oil turns unhealthy. For this reason, olive oil is not desirable to use for frying, because its smoke point is only 374 degrees. High smoke point oils such as coconut (446 degrees) and macadamia nut (392 degrees) are our favorites when we occasionally sauté foods. Jay and I prefer never to fry or deep fat fry our foods because of how unhealthy they are. Dark containers keep the oils from oxidizing and going rancid. We recommend only the following oils be used to assure maximum digestion, health and flavor:

Extra Virgin Olive Oil

in a dark glass or tin container, unrefined, organic, unheated.

Macadamia Nut Oil

Dark container and unrefined, unheated, unprocessed and organic.

Grape seed Oil

In a dark tin container or dark green glass container unprocessed, unheated , unrefined, organic

Refrigerated Flax/ Omega 3 seed oils

or a combination of flax and borage oils, contained in dark brown bottles, located in the refrigerated section of your local health food grocery store.

If you have been using Canola oil or peanut oil, we recommend you toss them out. Canola oils are man made. There is a very strong public relations company promoting a favorable marketing story about Canola oils because they have been paid to do so by the manufacturing companies. Jay and I do not recommend consumption of Canola oil, corn oil, peanut oil, Crisco oil, lard, or other "vegetable" oils found in grocery stores in plastic, clear containers.

Typically, they have been highly heated and over-processed, causing our bodies to have to break down these oils at temperatures higher than 450 degrees. Our bodies are only designed to have a natural temperature of 98.6 degrees. How can we digest and process oils heated at these temperatures? We can't; it is best not to ingest them at all.

Here are some more exotic oils you will enjoy trying, as we love them:

Pumpkinseed Oil is a pleasant, nutty-sweet oil which makes salads taste exceptionally good. The oil-rich pumpkinseed has a high protein content and was once a staple of ancient Aztecan and Mayan diets. Nutritionally, unrefined pumpkinseed oil is a highly prized and valuable whole food as well as an effective nutraceutical, as long as it is extracted in an unrefined, expeller pressed manner. Pumpkinseed oil can aid those who suffer from bladder weakness or incontinence, and it has long been reputed to prevent prostate enlargement.

This is a delicate oil and, as such, should only be used cold or drizzled over a cooked meal. It is best to purchase pumpkinseed oil in a dark container and keep it refrigerated.

Walnut Oil has been used for more than one thousand years. It is rich in linoleic acid (Omega-6), which produces prostaglandins.

Flax Oil

Flax Oil is in a class of its own because it is the only oil composed almost entirely of good poly-unsaturated, essential fatty acids. Essential fatty acids are those required by the body to sustain health. These fatty acids must come from food sources because the body cannot produce them. This oil goes rancid quickly and, therefore, needs to be refrigerated at all times. Not all manufacturers offer well-produced flax oil. Labels often read "cold-pressed" or "expeller-pressed," hiding the fact that the oil may have been refined after extraction. No legislation is in place to make companies disclose that their product has been refined. That's why we only purchase oils from reputable people we trust.

It is better to purchase small amounts of flax seed oil because it does go rancid quickly, even if refrigerated. It is also sensitive to light and oxygen. We systematically go through our oils once a month and throw away any that are too old.

Use flax oil only in cold dishes such as salads and pâtés, in living soups, and over potato salads. Or drizzle it over cooked foods if they are not very hot.

Hemp Oil

Hemp Oil There has been much talk recently about the power of hemp oil, simply because it is a nutritious oil with an excellent balance of essential fatty acids. Some nutritionists claim that the ratio between linoleic acid (Omega-3) and linoleic acid (Omega- 6) is nothing short of ideal. Hemp oil even contains the rare gamma-linoleic acid (GLA). Udo Erasmus, author of Fats That Heal, Fats That Kill, calls it the twin sister of flax oil because it shares the same health claims.

Unrefined, cold-pressed hemp oil has a fresh, nutty flavor. Like pumpkinseed and walnut oils, hemp oil should not be heated. Use it cold on baked potatoes and salads.

It is wise to read the label before purchasing. European importers often refine this oil, which results in a bland flavor, light color, and fair amounts of trans-fatty acids. Walnut oil contains a rich, nutty taste that is delicious in salads and can be poured over steamed vegetables. Like pumpkinseed oil, this oil must not be cooked but rather used cold or drizzled over cooked food.

Macadamia nuts are native to Australia and are rightfully called the queen of the nuts. Macadamia nut oil is heat stable. Like avocado oil, it has a long shelf life because it consists of mostly mono-unsaturated and saturated fatty acids, which do not go rancid easily. This oil adds a fine, nutty flavor to many hot dishes. If we have to stir-fry any veggies, this or coconut oil is our oil of choice, since its smoke temperature is higher than average.

Coconut Oil

Coconut Oil is 90 percent saturated fatty acids, however, these are lauric, myristic and palmitic fatty acids, which have low melting points. This is important because most of the saturates in this oil are in the form of medium chain triglyceride (MCTS), which are easily digested and not stored in the body as fat. In other words, you will not gain weight by eating coconut oil. Jay and I use coconut oil (unprocessed and unfiltered, organic) when we cook foods. Either macadamia or coconut oils will ONLY be used, because their smoke temperatures reach higher than 400 degrees. We never cook our foods that high, so we are safe; you will be, too, when you cook your foods this way. Other good fatty acids in coconut oil are 7.5 percent monounsaturated oleic fatty acids and 2.5 percent poly-unsaturated linoleic fatty acids.

Processing coconut oil the old fashioned, healthy way takes manufacturers a lot of time, so we suggest you purchase coconut oils only from the most reputable companies.

“Change your Kitchen

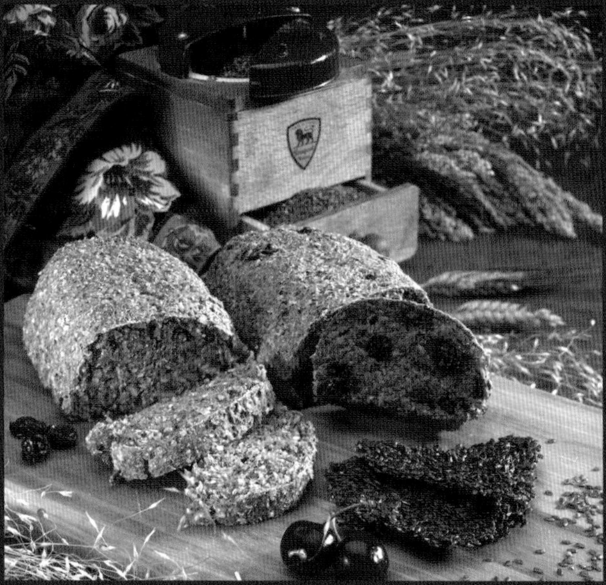

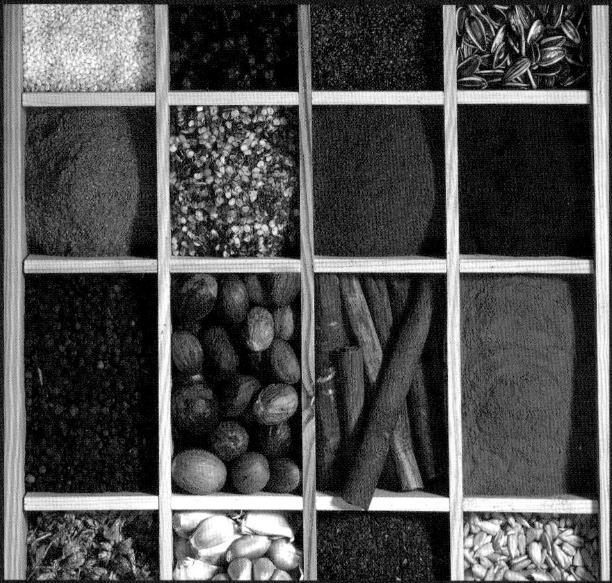

Change your Life"

Linda Kordich

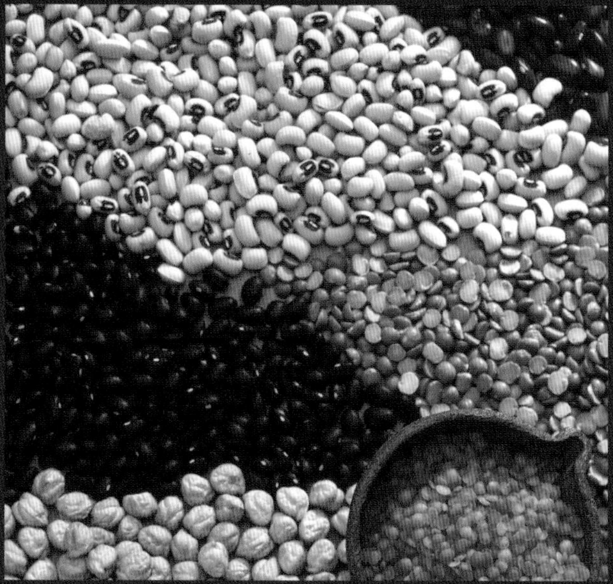

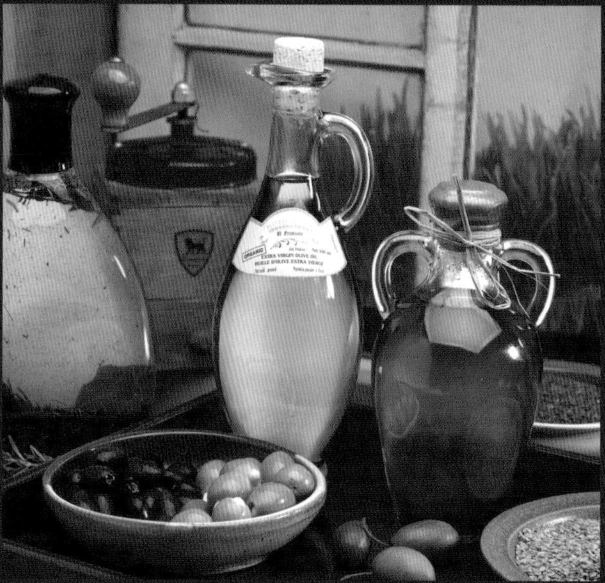

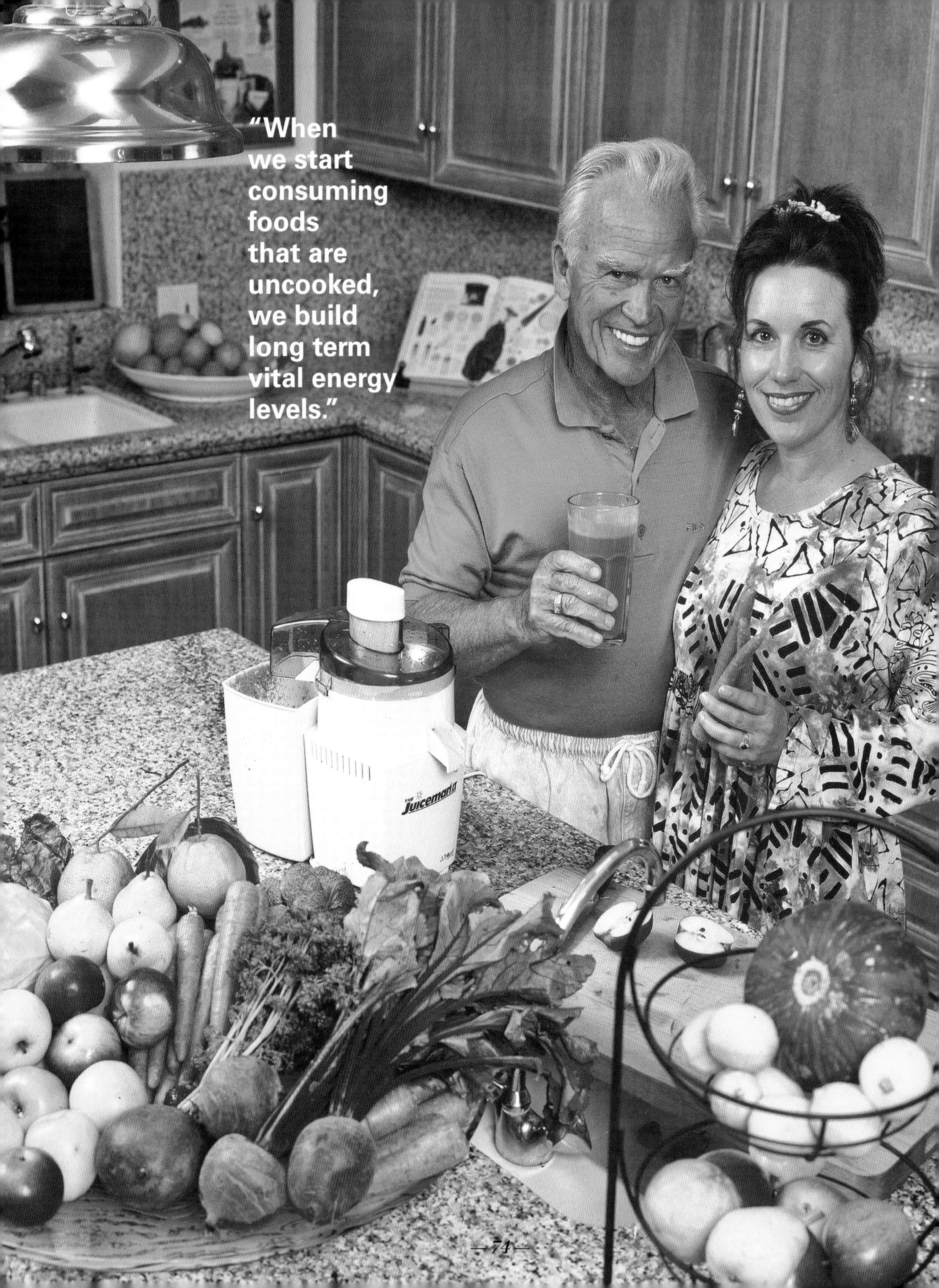

"When we start consuming foods that are uncooked, we build long term vital energy levels."

Chapter 6

Our Living Kitchen

- How to Create your own Living Kitchen
- Kitchen Appliances, Tools, and Organization
- Foods to Keep and Foods to Trash
- Let's go Shopping the The Live Foods Live Bodies way
- Taking an Esoteric Approach to Our Living Kitchen

Our Live Foods Live Bodies Program is our full spectrum approach to foods that embrace our Mind, Body, *and Heart.*

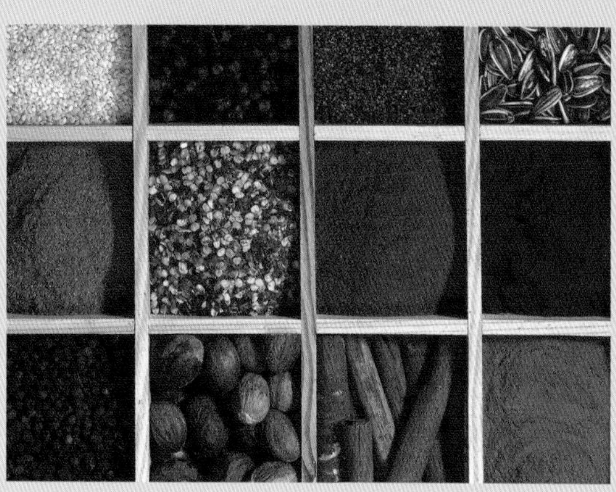

When we consume primarily living foods, our bodies feel more alive, which in turn ignites our own state of well-being. In order to live a disease-free lifestyle, it's not just the foods we choose. There are other aspects we must respect and integrate to sustain this sacred, long-living type of lifestyle. Our program will help you and your loved ones build a harmonious outlook toward true nourishment in what we've lovingly come to call Our Living Kitchen. Our next book, entitled Our Living Kitchen goes into great depth on issues we are only touching on now. There's so much to say, that Jay and I decided we wanted to lay the foundation of this book, Live Foods Live bodies, first.

Our Living Kitchen

Our Living Kitchen philosophy helps redefine how we think and feel about food, our kitchen, appliances and our attitudes towards all of them. For example, you will learn to prepare delicious meals in ten minutes or less. You will discover new, supportive appliances and tools few people know about, but you will especially enjoy the changing relationship you will start to develop between you and your kitchen. When we start consuming foods from Nature, we keep our vital energy protected by eating more and more living foods. Moreover, Nature returns to us the gift of not only great cellular health, but she will start to evolve throughout our hearts, ultimately instilling in us a deep sense and reverence and respect for living foods, animals, ourselves and others. Within time, our lives and the lives we touch change on many levels. How can this be? Because when we start to hook into the healing aspects of nature, animals, and living foods, we somehow start to change from the inside out.

giving us an understanding about life that is priceless and everlasting. However, before we get into it let me give you a brief summary of our personal history of how we came about such a wonderful, empowering lifestyle.

How it all got Started

Without consciously realizing it, the evolution of Our Living Kitchen actually started back in our childhoods. Jay and I were both raised by European parents. Even though Jay was born in 1923 and I was born in 1955, my grandparents were born in the same years as his parents. My grandparents reared me until I was thirteen. Fortunately for

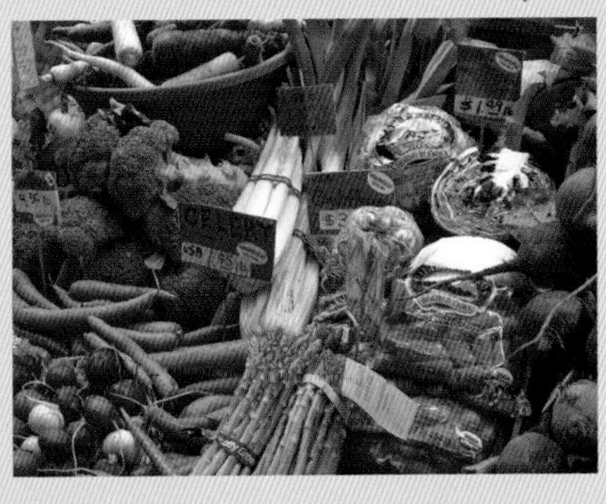

me, my grandmother was head chef for a prestigious hotel in Norway before she migrated to America, and as a result, she became the head of our family kitchen, preparing outstanding meals every night.

Luckily, both of our families cultivated rich, lush gardens throughout the year—which our neighbors back then strangely considered backwards. But to us, homemade black breads, natural meals, and gardens were the norm, and they were something to feel quite proud about. Jay and I enjoyed personal experiences with growing, picking, and helping to prepare naturally fully ripened foods daily. What we didn't realize then was that this process became a rich, and soul-rewarding way of eating, something for which I am very grateful for learning at such a young age. It's interesting that both my grandparents and Jay's parents are now gone, yet we think of them daily, integrating so much they have taught to us, so that we may now teach others.

Even if you don't have a grandparent or parent to teach you how to garden, you can find someone to mentor you. Take a class, talk to a neighbor, or purchase a good book on organic gardening. I highly recommend gardening to enhance your Living Foods experience, even if done minimally with a few garden pots on a balcony or patio. Gardening can influence your life because it is a direct link to beauty and to the mystery of nature. As your plants blossom, within time so will your relationship with food, your connection to food and nature, and your connection with your own personal experiences in your kitchen. After all, this is where we either find ourselves in states of frustration or creativity.

Like Your Kitchen?

How comfortable do you feel in your kitchen? Do you feel empowered, and in control of your family's health needs, as well as your own? In reality, most of us don't. Mostly, we actually feel daunted by the responsibilities imposed upon us by our families and our desire to capture vital health, yet it's truly my belief that we want to feel connected, yet we just don't know how to go about doing it. We also feel it will take way too much time to learn. This is true in a way, because everywhere we turn, in the real world, we get zero support when it comes to learning and integrating these noble types of lifestyles.

. Grocery stores dedicate 85 percent of their shelf space to packaged, canned, and prepared foods. They are cheap to create yet are extremely costly in dollars and to our health. This dysfunctional way of eating only supports the pockets of the manufacturers and not your ability to nourish yourself and your family. As someone once said, "Stop the insanity!" Don't fret. We have the answer.

It may surprise you, but here is how it goes:

Simple Foods = Power Foods!

Universal truths are simple and short. If we simplify our natural foods selection in each meal we eat, they in turn become powerfully effective in our bodies. For example, a whole meal salad is all you need for a dinner. When did it become a law that we need a three-course dinner, or five different kinds of foods on our plate? When I was little, my grandmother made dinner every night, as you most likely have learned earlier in this chapter. But life was much more simple back then, and she was trained as a chef. Unfortunately, we are living in a different time, and the stress to perform is very high.

What we are finding out now is that green foods, salads with more than three different colored vegetables present, is where the real power is. We are finding through scientific research that fiber foods are power foods. Fiber is prolific

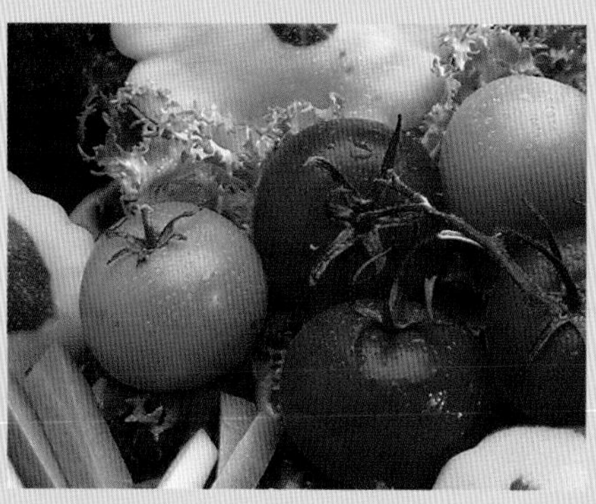

in salads. Researchers are also discovering that foods that are high in water content and bright in colors are especially important to humans. When you eat this way, you do not stress. Life is so much easier!

Which foods do you think have high water content in them? You guessed it—greens, fruits, and vegetables. The natural waters found in fruits are so powerful and healing that cosmetic manufacturers are now trying to encapsulate them because of their powerful healing effects on the skin. But why should we pay three hundred times the cost? Why not just go directly to nature and consume these wonderful foods?

I guess my personal opinion is that most of us don't have a personal relationship with natural foods. This may sound corny but there's so much truth to this statement. This is one of the reasons Jay and I decided to write this book. Once we trust, then we can learn in a way that is long term, especially when you can connect with great resources.

Below you will find lifestyle change that will help you change from poor habits to empowering habits.

TIPS FOR VITALITY

- Try to eat a rainbow of different colors from fruits and vegetables daily.
- Try to eat high-water content foods (fruits, greens, vegetables) daily.
- Try to eat at least up to one pound of salad per day.
- Try to juice at least twenty-four ounces of vegetable daily.
- Try to exercise forty minutes per day, especially outdoors.
- Get sun twenty minutes per day between 10-11am or 2-3pm
- Try to pray every day for grace, mercy, peace, forgiveness, understanding and how to lead a virtuous life
- Try to drink at least six to eight, eight-ounce glasses of steam-distilled water daily (not including the juice).
- When you eat grains or beans, soak them for twenty-four hours beforehand.
- Give time to a charity, or help an older neighbor or grandchild weekly.

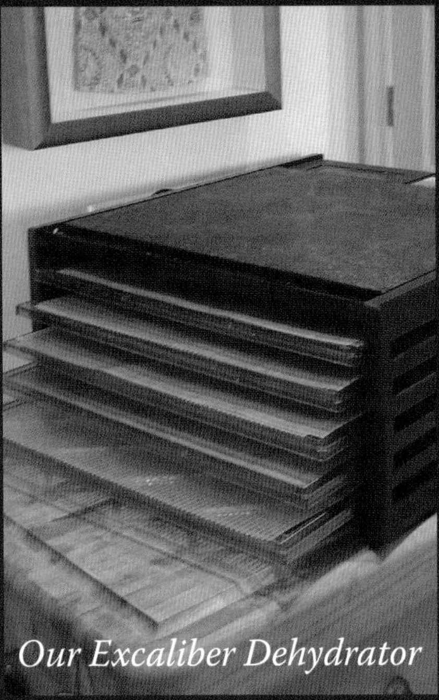

Our Excaliber Dehydrator

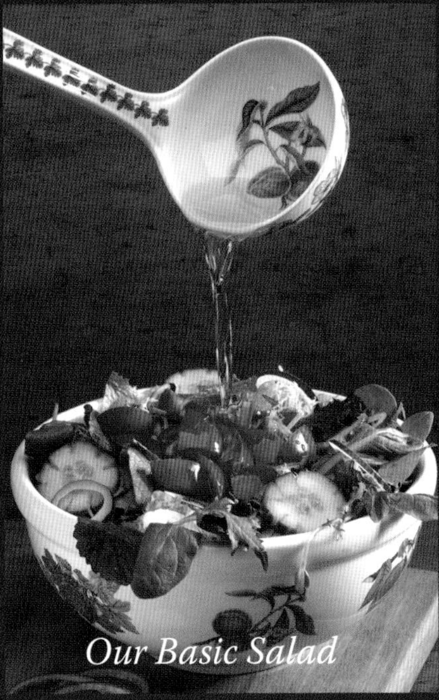

Our Basic Salad

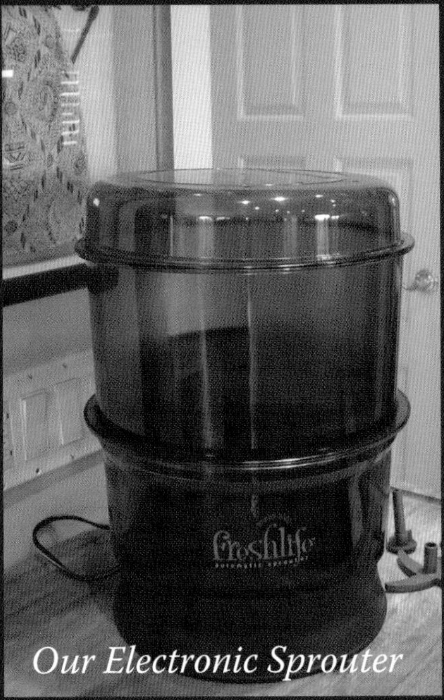

Our Electronic Sprouter

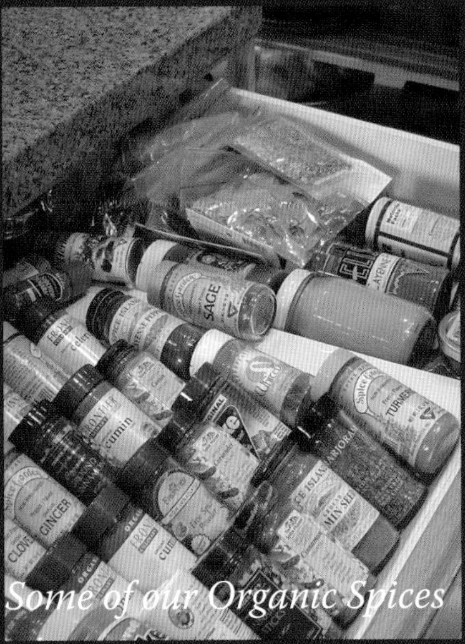

Some of our Organic Spices

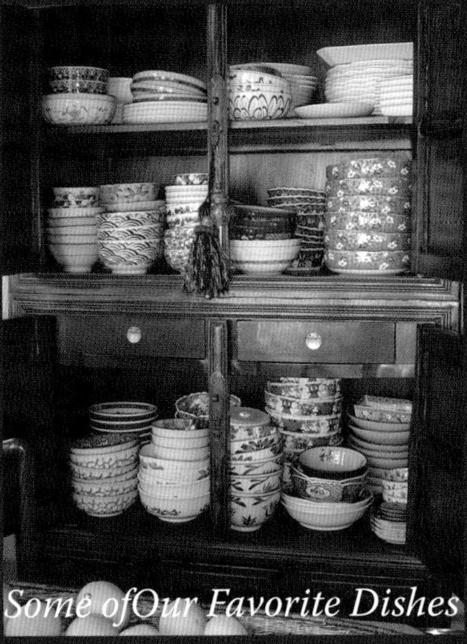

Some ofOur Favorite Dishes

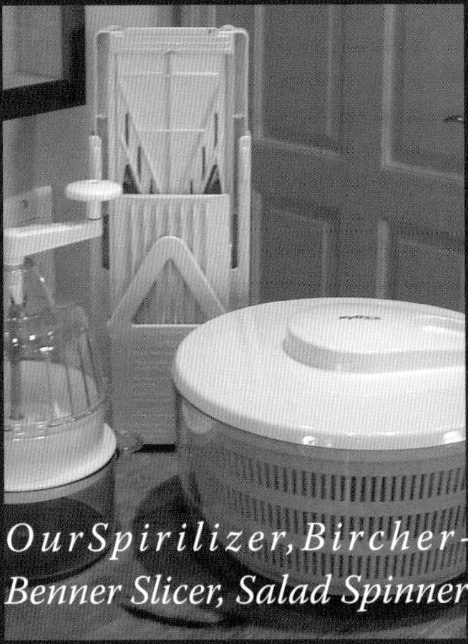

OurSpirilizer,Bircher-Benner Slicer, Salad Spinner

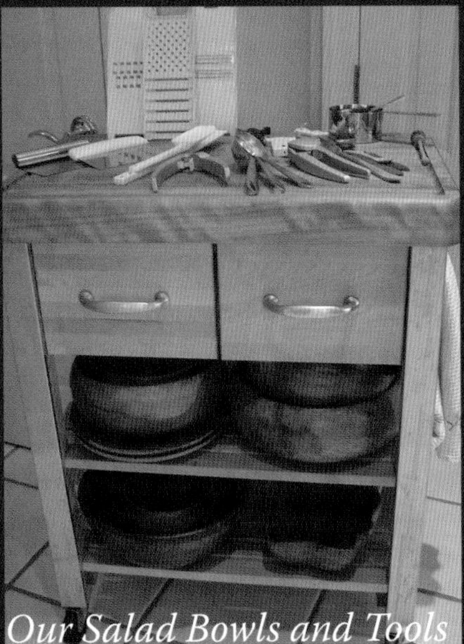

Our Salad Bowls and Tools

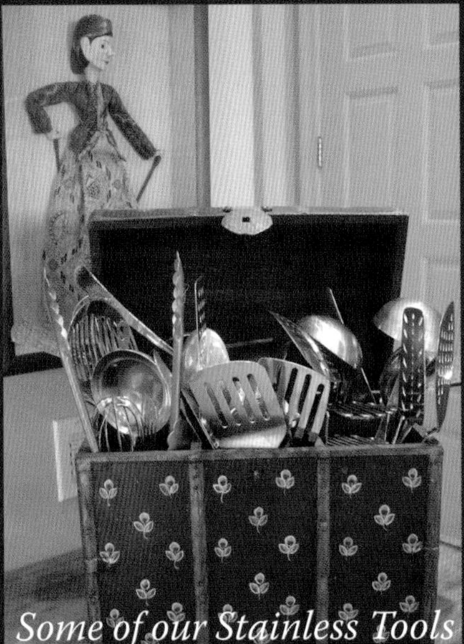

Some of our Stainless Tools

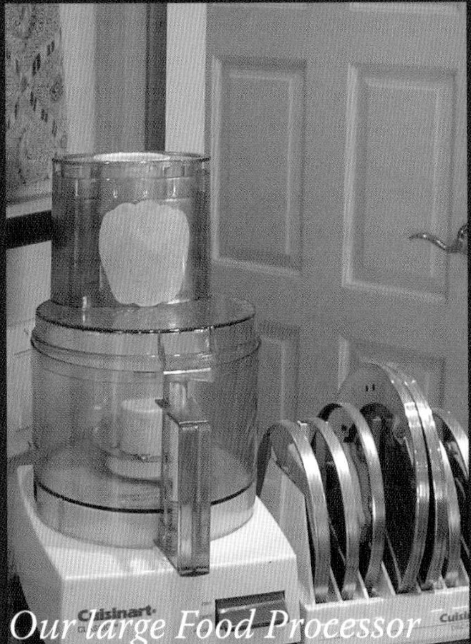

Our large Food Processor

What does Our Living Kitchen look like?

Because of Jay's high profile in America for so many years, our neighbors would invariably ask us what steps they could make to improve their diets.

Ultimately, this took us into their kitchens. What we found interesting was that their kitchens, pantries, and refrigerators looked completely different from ours. (Jay and I lived for so many years in our own natural foods world, that we were somewhat shocked to see how typical American families lived and ate.) Placed on the counter tops of their kitchens, we saw coffee makers, microwave ovens, Teflon-coated cookware, aluminum cookware and bake ware, deep-fat fryers, electric can openers, and Teflon-coated utensils, amongst a myriad of other mysterious looking plastic coated tools.

Our Friends' Kitchen looked very different from Ours

Their pantries were filled to the top with canned, packaged, and processed foods. What really took us aback was the sea of different colored canned sodas lurking in the cabinets. Cereals loaded with artificial colors, sugars, and additives dominated the shelves, too. If that weren't bad enough, a full complement of hydrogenated oil-laden snack foods lay in wait. When we saw the Crisco oil, we realized they were in deep trouble. This is when we realized wealth did not equal food intelligence. We knew our advice was going to be disconcerting, so we tried to be gentle with our comments.

What better way than to show them our kitchen? Somewhat foreign to them, our counter tops displayed products they were not very familiar with, such as our professional juicer, high-powered blender, food processor, dehydrator, electric tea pot, steam distiller, bamboo steamer, and multi-grain rice cooker. (Our complete list is on page 82). We further satisfied their curiosity when we opened the refrigerator. In our bins, we had carrots, already cut up and ready for juicing; bags of washed greens and vegetables, ready for salads; glass containers filled with sprouted grains; soaked nuts or pâtés ready for the next meal; freshly made almond milk; very few bottled food jars; and some health-food type junk food for one of our yet unenlightened teenage sons! Shocked that the fruit bin held only apples and no other fruits, our friends were surprised to see so much fruit displayed on the counters. We explained that when fruit is made available in this way, its fragrance and beauty inspire us (and, we hope, our children) to eat it abundantly throughout the day.

Touring the kitchen had to include not just the refrigerator and appliances, but the pantry as well. At the bottom of our pantry, we kept vegetables such as onions and potatoes in separate bins. In the middle of the shelves aromatic scents from our dried herbs and spices seemed to dominate our senses. And our green, black, white, and herbal teas from around the world offered their own unique fragrances. We also had a small amount of canned foods which we use very sparingly. We probably spend about $50.00 per month on foods such as bottled mustards, relishes, organic oils, sesame tahini and nut butters. (see more on page 64-65 and page 83)

As we mentioned before, our youngest son is still in process of evolving toward a purer diet. Even though he likes some junk food, he only consumes natural sodas and cereals, and some borderline products. Luckily, he is a self-committed vegetarian who eats close to 50 percent living foods and juices daily, so the only challenges we have with him are with the "fun" foods. Jay and I are confident he will learn to balance his food choices at his own comfort level and in his own good time.

Peer pressure issues have a great impact on children. As with anything in life, children deserve the same respect as adults, especially when it comes to making life-altering changes. As healthfully as Jay and I both eat and inspire others to do, and as much as we would like our children to follow our eating regimes, we can't expect our children to be just like us. We try to show our children by example, which we believe is the best long-term way to teach.

The advice we gave our friends about their diets tended to suggest the same, simple course of action each time. You, too, can now be empowered by these very same steps you will shortly learn in our program.

Our Living Kitchen principles are presented with two aspects in mind: The first part is practical, where you will look at your pantry, refrigerator, food choices, kitchen appliances, and tools to help build your own Living Kitchen. The other part is more esoteric and fun. You will discover what's been missing in your approach to the kitchen and how powerful changing your diet can be. Plus, you'll get to try our rich variety of recipes to introduce you to a new way of eating.

How to Quick-Start Your Own Living Kitchen

Jay and I love our kitchen. That's because everything we need—knives, bowls, appliances, kitchen tools, herbs, and spices—is right at our fingertips. When our kitchen is organized efficiently, we enjoy maximum function of our tools and appliances as well as the ability to quickly prepare ready-to-use produce. More importantly, our kitchen is set up to display and store only those tools and appliances that support our healthy eating style. Similarly, the only foods we buy and store are those that support the kind of healthful meal preparation we desire to maintain. As you read further, you will see how this makes all the difference in making the preparation of living and natural foods a pleasurable experience. Once you learn to adopt Our Living Kitchen principles, you will love your kitchen too.

STEP 1: The Kitchen Clean-Out

To turn your kitchen into your own Living Kitchen typically requires a few adjustments and

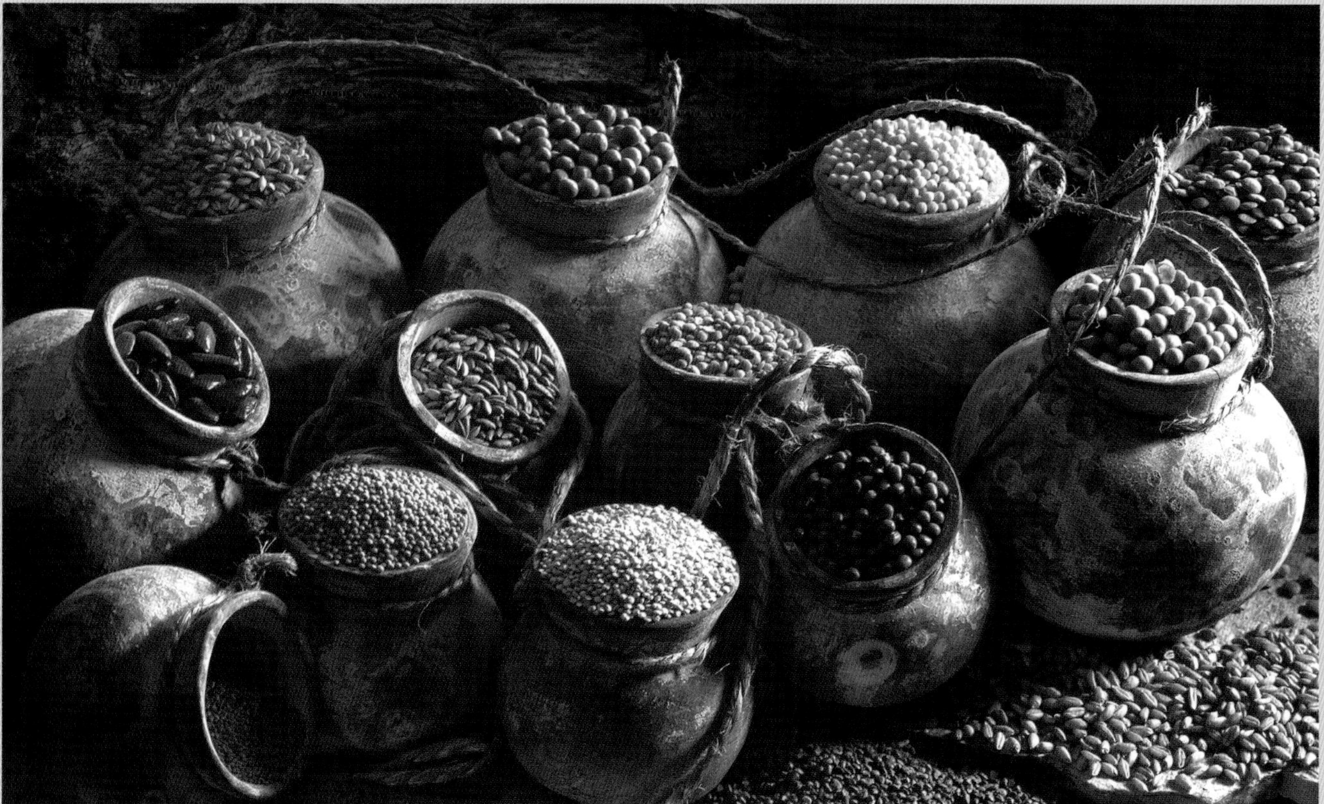

considerations. It's best to begin with an overall kitchen clean out. This is what I've learned to do which helps everything go faster, and be more enjoyable.

- Dedicate three hours of your time to this project
- Turn on some inspiring music
- Change into comfortable clothes
- Light a candle to help change the atmosphere
(Remember to blow it out when you are finished)

Here's a check list to help you evaluate what simple or gradual changes you can make in setting up your ownLiving Kitchen. Yes, this is a must. You will be grateful when it's over. To begin a new you and new family, cleaning out the old not only is a great practical idea, it's a metaphysical one too. To become new in spirit and alive with this new energy coming into your home, we must think that the old energy of you must leave. Don't get discouraged. Just take it a step at a time, if it seems too burdensome or overwhelming. If you get overwhelmed and need help, if you have children, ask them! They may balk at first, but trust me, they will appreciate the experience, and it anchors them to having more awareness about kitchen organization and how much time and dedication it takes to keep things organized and beautiful.

1. Evaluate Your Appliances and Tools

Look at the appliances and tools in your present kitchen and ask yourself if each item supports living health or undermines your ability to become healthier. The ten items listed below have been deemed suspect, over time, in undermining our ability to stay healthy. You can peruse www.Google.com on the Internet to find more enlightening information that will guide you to learn what Jay and I have researched and have known for many years about the possible health risks in using these types of appliances. It's our belief, Aluminum cookware and Teflon coated utensils, tools and appliances are partly responsible for kidney stone formation, tumors, along with Alzheimer's Disease. It's sad to see manufactures here in America create cookware, appliances and kitchen tools that can be so harmful to our health. To make matters worse, they sell these appliances to third world countries who do not have the intelligence or information to know the difference. Only a small percentage of Americans are informed, yet Jay and I are working hard, to bring to light, these controversies and major concerns we have about toxic coated cookware.

It is wise to discontinue using the following unhealthy tools and Appliances:

Poor Kitchen Appliances (Not Recommended for a Healthy Lifestyle)	
Aluminum Cookware	Deep-fat Fryers of any kind
Non-stick Cookware of all kinds	Coffee makers
Dishes containing Lead	Teflon-coated Frying pans
Teflon-coated Cookware and Utensils/Tools	Rotisseries and/or Roasters
Pottery Cookware	Grills, Aluminum or Teflon coated
Microwave Ovens	Barbecues of all kinds
Anodized Aluminum Cookware	Microwavable Plastic Cookware of any kind

We suggest, for those on a budget, to remember that we put the appliances and tools in order of importance so you can add them gradually to your kitchen. Sometimes you can find these appliances gently used, either through eBay or through want ads. If you're a lucky newlywed, you may want to include these on your registry. If you are a parent with children who are newlyweds, we suggest you help them build their own Living Kitchen through time.

Tools and Appliances used in Our Living Kitchen	
1. Professional Juice Extractor	14. Salad Spinner (for greens)
2. Professional High powered Blender	15. Cheesecloth for straining nut milks
3. Wheatgrass Juicer (stainless only)	16. Saladaccio (for spiralizing veggies)
4. Professional grade Knives	17. Boerner Slicer (and variations thereof)
5. Paring Knife (for citrus)	18. Pyrex or similar for food storage
6. Food Processor (large)	19. Large glass containers for Suntea. (1/2 gal.)
7. Food Processor (small for dressings)	20. Glass jars (1 pint) for storage of dressings/
8. Electric Teapot	pate's and sauces/and/or sprouts/soaked nuts
9. Steam distiller or Steamed distilled water	20. Soymilk Maker (Automatic)
10. Automatic Sprouter (see page 78 for picture)	21 Tofu Maker (hand or machine)
11. Dehydrator (not to exceed 120 degrees)	22. Stainless Steel Cookware 100% 18/10
12. Electronic Pesticide wash remover	23. Pressure Cooker (stainless steel)
13. Nut and Seed Grinder	24. Stainless Steel Wok (for steaming veggies)

You may go to our website www.JayKordich.com to see our personal appliances and appliances we recommend.

2. Consider your foods carefully

Cleaning out your kitchen cabinets, pantry, and refrigerator gives you an opportunity to be mindful about the kinds of foods you really do want in your kitchen for nourishing yourself and your family. Begin by looking at food labels and eliminating anything on the Worst Foods to Eat list that follows. Also, check for foods you haven't used in the past year, such as packaged foods, canned foods, spices and herbs. Remember, anything in a jar or packaged is not living, so therefore, like we do, keep your pantry to a minimum. On the next page you will find acceptable foods we find to be helpful in the preparation of our Live foods Live Bodies Program.

Whatever you get rid of could be offered to a food shelter or relegated to storage for a while if you are hard-pressed to part with certain items. It's crucial to makes these changes. Why? Because when you are clear of clutter and foods that do not support your own vital health, you will then have room to store new tools and foods that *do* support vibrant living health. On the following page, you will find foods we recommend to eliminate. They are not in order of importance.

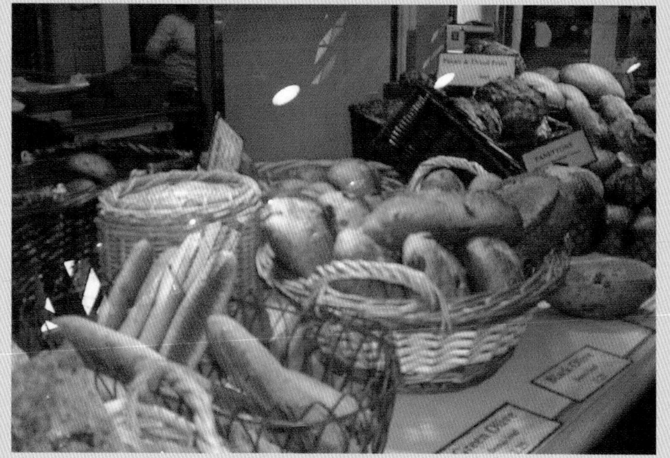

Recommended foods to be eliminated:

- Foods containing hydrogenated or partially hydrogenated oils (especially found in almost all snack foods like crackers, chips, cookies, muffins, cakes, pies, candy bars, cereals, coffee creamers, and most prepared mixes)
- Saturated fats such as Crisco, lard, and margarine
- Heat extracted oils, including cottonseed oils, safflower oils, corn oil and peanut oil in plastic, clear bottles
- Foods containing artificial colors and flavors

.Foods containing artificial sweeteners

- Deli meats containing nitrates and nitrites
- White sugar products
- White flour products
- White rice (even white basmati rice)
- . All breads containing dough conditioners/calcium proprionate, mono diglycerides,and especially yeast. (Brewer's yeast is acceptable)
- Dairy products, unless unpasteurized and organic
- Artificially flavored and colored soft drinks
- Coffees of all kinds
- All Alcohol, including wines containing sulfur dioxide and those made from non-organic grapes
- All carbonated sodas

Here is a list of packaged foods we keep in our refrigerator:

- Bottled organic Relish
- Bottled organic Sauerkraut
- Bottled nut Butters
- Bottled natural organic Mayonnaise
- Bottled organic Oils for our salads
- Bottled organic Ketchup
- Bottled organic prepared Mustards
- Packaged Teas
- Packaged Herbs, Spices and Condiments. (Please read all labels-organic)
- Packaged Organic Tofu (refrigerated types).
- Sesame Tahini (organic)

3. Here are some important tips for setting up your new Living Kitchen:

- Organize dried herbs and spices close to your food preparation area, but in a cool, dark place, since heat can affect their taste and quality.
- Store oils such as borage or flax in the refrigerator, and others in a dark area away from heat, as heat causes the oils to go rancid.
- Nuts, being rich in essential fats and oils, go rancid in time at room temperature, so keep them in the refrigerator.

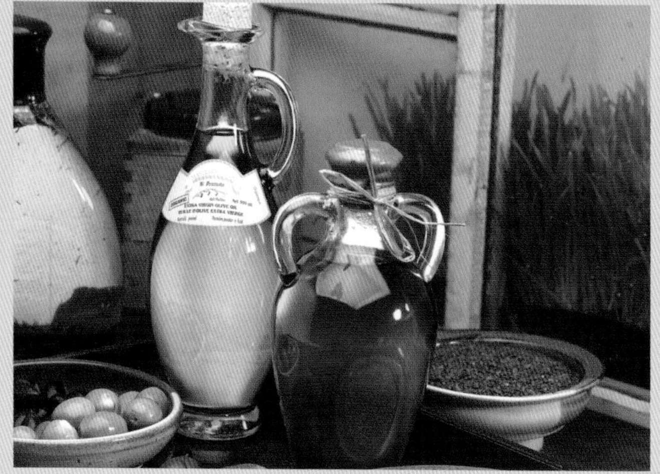

If you have an abundance of measuring cups, bowls, spoons, and storage containers, always keep the glass ones over plastic. (Tupperware is not something we recommend, but if you like it and have lots of it, keep it. Just refrain from putting either fresh fruit or very hot foods inside plastic containers. Jay and I have slowly collected Pyrex glass lidded containers, which we find are more sterile and functional.)

Our Living Kitchen Principles to Remember:

1. **Does this tool or appliance support my ability to create living foods for myself and your family?**
2. **Be wise with the foods you bring home. Remember, whatever you bring home is a temptation.**
3. **Rethink the amount of fresh/living foods you eat. Whenever you eat a meal, ask yourself "How much of my food is living?" The ideal should be: (At least 50-70%)**

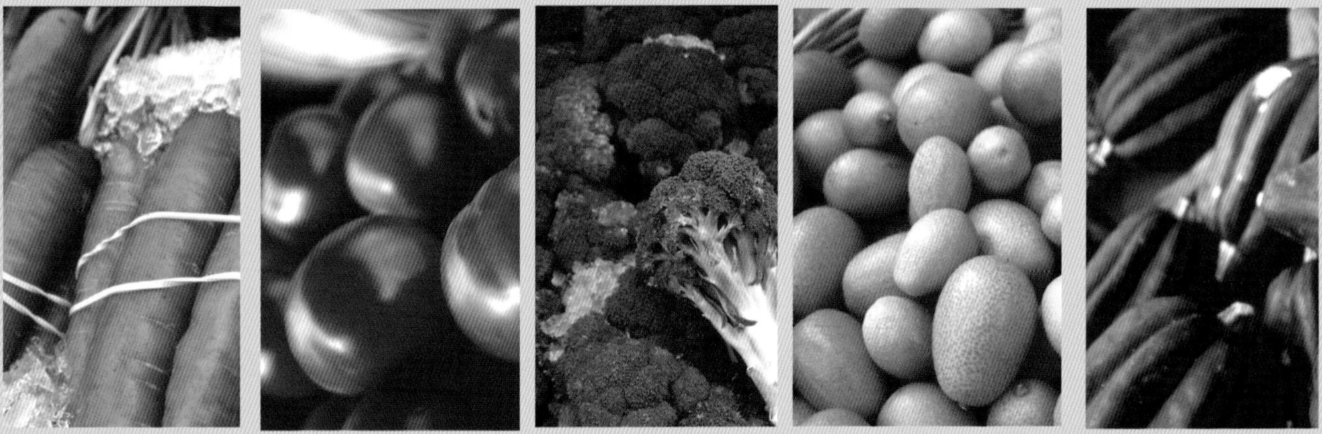

Now that you have modified and enhanced the structure of your new kitchen, it's time to have fun filling it with the choicest ingredients possible to support your wonderful, new health style. Jay and I invite you into our kitchen to show you what we do when we come home from the grocery store.

Let's Go Grocery Shopping - With Living Foods!

Jay and I have developed an Our Living Kitchen food-shopping system that works really well for us. We go to the grocery store twice a week. (See page 105) On Fridays, we purchase all the foods we'll use for the next several days, along with a twenty-five pound bag of "organic horse carrots," from our local grocer. (These carrots are much less expensive in bulk and are nice big, sweet carrots. In fact, we purchase them for $4.99 for the entire twenty-five pound bag). We make sure we buy enough grains (either for sprouting or cooking), apples, avocados, and fresh vegetables and fruits to accommodate our sons' friends who often spend the weekend.

On Wednesdays, we go to the farmer's market close to our home. This is where we buy really great organic greens for our salads and what's in season regarding vegetables and fruits. We usually buy about four different kinds of vegetables and four different kinds of fruits every week. Mid-week, we also purchase additional fresh

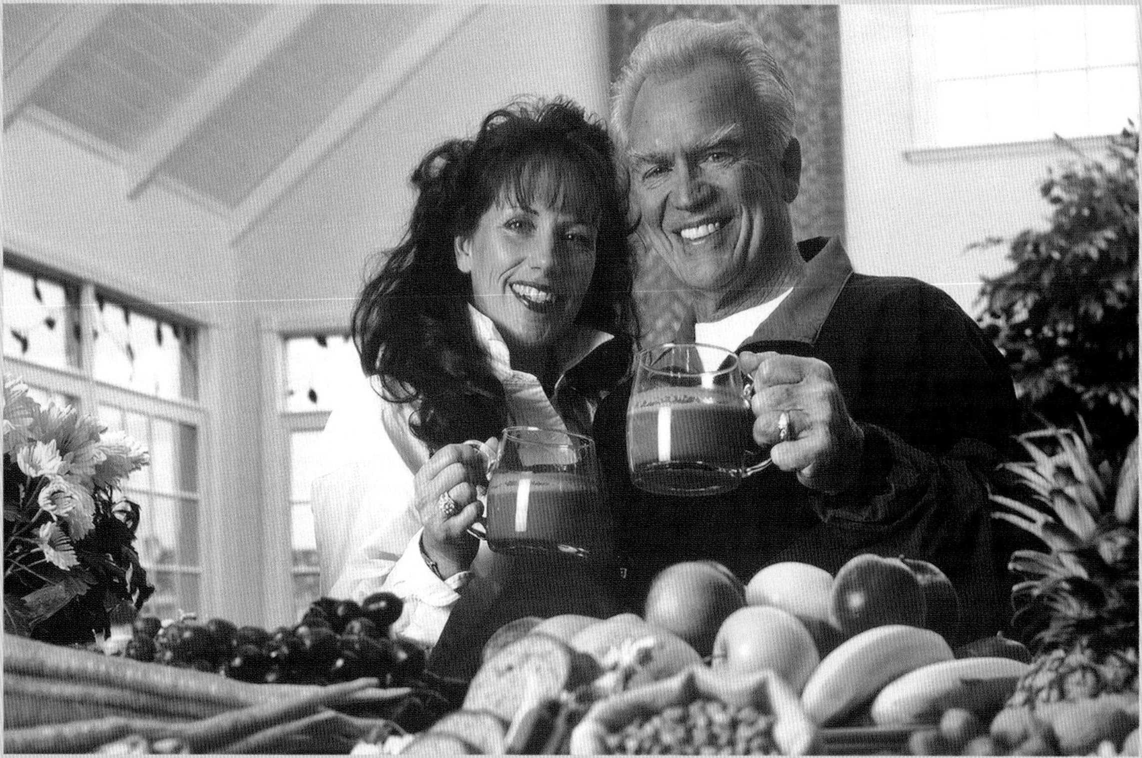

fruits and vegetables (that stay in keeping with the four veggies and four fruits) as well as staples such as olive oils, flax seed, and nuts. It's ideal to cycle in vegetables and fruits throughout the week so that everything doesn't ripen simultaneously and then spoil if not used.

What's Next?

Once home from the grocery store, Jay immediately washes the carrots. I change into sweats or something comfy, put Josh Groban, Yanni, or Enya on the stereo, light a candle, say an affirmation, and then take about thirty to forty-five minutes to clean all the produce. We always try to buy organic produce, and when we can't, we use a produce wash designed to clean and remove pesticide residues. (You can go to our Web site, www.jaykordich.com) for a wonderful pesticide wash we created for ourselves that is now available to the public.) We wash everything with water in one sink and use the other sink (or a bucket) for rinsing. Fruits and vegetables with water-resistant skins like apples, plums, and tomatoes, are best washed at this time, too. But delicate produce like berries, peaches, kiwi, and mushrooms are best washed right before eating or juicing.

We Partner Together in the Kitchen

I wash the greens, spin-dry them, and put them in a plastic zipper lock bag for the fridge. ready for either salad preparation or juicing. If you are not fond of washing, spin-drying, and storing greens, Jay and I often purchase a product we happily recommend called Evolution Organic Baby Field Greens. When we are prepared to eat or juice, we are ready to go at any time. Juicing and salad preparation now only takes a few minutes. These greens come already washed and bagged, and they last up to four days after opening. In other cases, such as purchasing individual greens such as parsley, cilantro, or spinach, we spin-dry them thoroughly. Since even the smallest amount of water can turn the leaves brown and mushy if not consumed in a few days, we layer an absorbent paper towel into bagged greens of all kinds to really help extend their freshness.

Before putting the veggies into the fridge, I check for produce that has been overlooked and going bad. We generally keep fruits on the counter, although we do refrigerate apples and berries to preserve their freshness.

It is best to preserve berries in an airtight container (preferably glass, because fruit acids leach into the plastic when placed together). We also wrap fresh berries in a paper towel before we place them into the container.

Pressure Free for the Rest of the Week

When we finish the washing process, we feel absolutely free of pressure. Knowing our refrigerator is now stocked with ready-to-use produce means we are able to approach mealtimes quickly and effortlessly. By now, Jay has his carrots all washed, trimmed, and prepared for juicing, and now I'm relaxed knowing that the salad and meal preparation for the upcoming week will be a breeze. While fresh is always best, sometimes busy schedules dictate that we purchase frozen, organic fruits (in season, unsweetened, and flash-frozen, for smoothies only) and we usually buy pre-washed, bagged, organic items such as salad greens. From start to finish, this process takes about 30 minutes.

After the produce is cleaned and stored, I may make organic brown rice with our stainless steel rice maker that will last us up to five days. However, whenever we make a grain for cooking, we always soak our grains at least six hours or overnight before we cook them. (This enhances their enzymatic ability to help us digest our foods better.) Then I will also decide to prepare a soup from any veggies going soft in the fridge

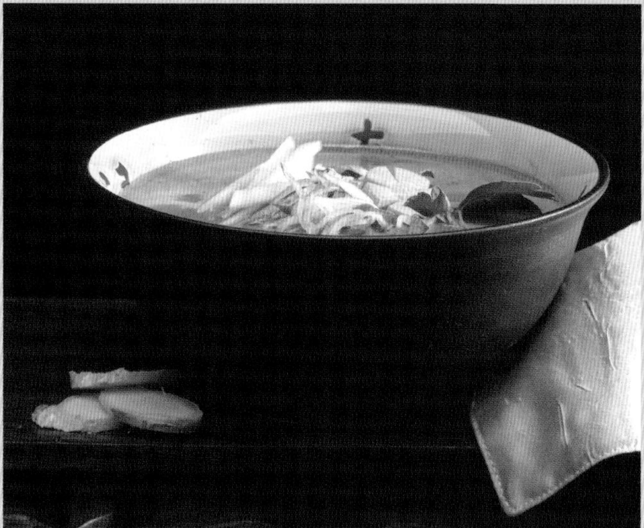

that should last about five days. Even though some of our soups are cooked, they offer their place in our diet. Jay and I are predominately living foodists, but in the winter, we eat about 25-30% of our meal with cooked grains or soups.

If you do this program twice a week and follow this style of advance preparation, making meals is incredibly easy and joyful. Trust me, it works. I have always been fascinated with people who think natural foods are complex and time-consuming. On the contrary, I find heavily cooked, meat-based meals take much more time and effort. When you try it our way, you will be absolutely amazed. The biggest benefit to this regime is the ability that, at any time, you have everything ready to prepare a great meal within ten-fifteen minutes.

The Heart and Soul of Our Living Kitchen

Now that you know how Our Living Kitchen is set up and how we prepare the foods we take home, you know everything Jay and I do to prepare healthful meals. What is more difficult to convey is the loving feeling we have when we are in our kitchen preparing food. These feelings are behind the more esoteric, difficult-to-define, but beneficial reasons to create your own Living Kitchen.

The kitchen is synonymous with food and the source of primary human comfort, both physical and emotional. But not everyone experiences food with positive satisfaction or optimal health. When I was about seventeen years old, I deeply suffered with anorexia and bulimia. I endured this nightmare for almost ten years, ruining my entire digestive system and my teeth. Therefore, I have tremendous compassion for men and women who suffer not only from this disease, but from any kind of food addiction.

In my future book, entitled My Kitchen Sanctuary, I will share my entire experience in hopes of helping others understand that this disease can be cured. I introduce this issue briefly now because my dark past allows me to share an inner wisdom regarding pure foods and vital health that comes from years of long personal suffering. In the past, anxiety over food led me to view the kitchen with fear and trepidation, since it was a source of great emotional turmoil for me.

Honoring our Kitchen is Divine

Happily, over time, a new consciousness about food allowed me to regard the kitchen with a freeing sense of love and safety. This is why I honor our kitchen. My kitchen *is* my sanctuary. It is a place where I honor myself, the foods I choose for my family, and the supreme energy from something higher that surrounds and enriches me. But it took a long time of dedication, patience and therapy to help me transition from feeling imprisoned, to being and feeling liberated. Living foods are a great catalyst for removing any kind of addiction.

Put some "Life" into your Kitchen

When you decide to make your kitchen a place full of life, energy, and love, your life will change for the better, too. This super-consciousness is waiting for you. It isn't necessary to suffer like I did in order to appreciate how liberating being in your kitchen can be. All it requires is a change in perception. Disregard the popular view that the kitchen is a place of drudgery to hectically prepare a variety of frozen, microwavable trays of food day after day. Instead, try to open your heart to see your kitchen as your sanctuary rather than a prison. It is a place to honor the supreme energy evident in these sun-energized and nutrient-rich foods Mother Nature shares with us.

Hold fast to the idea that preparing meals filled with love and respect will nourish the body beyond the cellular level. Consuming these foods in their natural states as much as possible transmutes their life-giving properties into our bodies for our optimal physical and mental well-being. When viewing food in this way, we can develop a most gratifying feeling to have abundant access to it and be able to prepare and share it with family and friends. This feeling leads to preparing food with intention, attention, and love—all key ingredients for making truly delicious food, and I may add, truly delicious experiences.

Learning to Love Your Kitchen by Creating a Sacred Space

If thinking in these new terms is appealing to you, it may be easiest to adopt these concepts as your own by practicing some of the following before preparing a meal. Here are a few examples of what I did that led to rewarding eating changes in my life:

- **Light a Candle.**
- **Say an Affirmation.***
- **Put on Music that Soothes your Soul.**
- **Put a Picture next to the Candle of those you Love, even if it's your Pet.**
- **Try to grow Fresh Herbs in your Kitchen**

*An affirmation can be a few simple words, such as "I open my heart to new feelings about preparing food in my kitchen." This can be said once or repeated several times, aloud or silently, for greater effectiveness. If you prefer a more spiritual approach, I suggest you pray according to the religion of your choice. I like praying to the Supreme Father so as to encompass all religions. All religions and philosophies have one thing in common: to love God with all of our hearts and souls. Here is an affirmation I have used in the kitchen for many years:

"To the Supreme Father of Divine Light and Mercy, please help me see my kitchen as a holy sanctuary to not only nourish every cell in my body and in those whom I serve, but to instill Your divine love into every meal I prepare. For this opportunity, I am *deeply* grateful."

"Simple Foods are

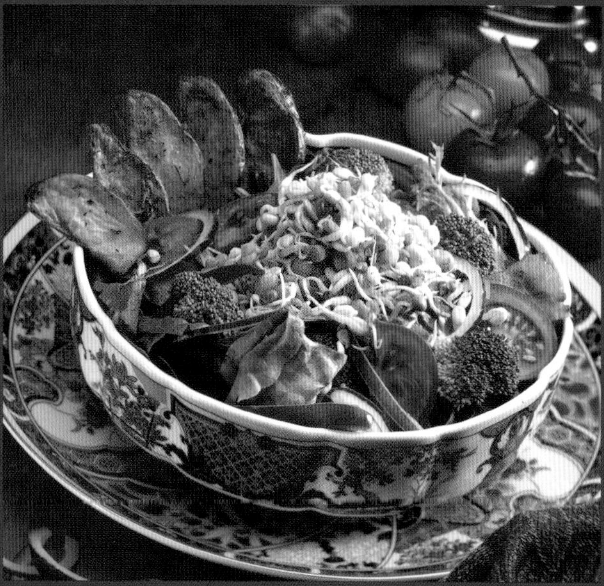

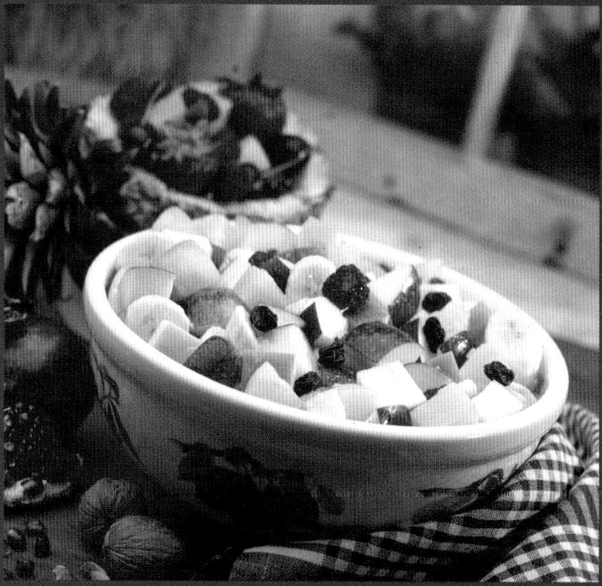

Power Foods"

Jay Kordich

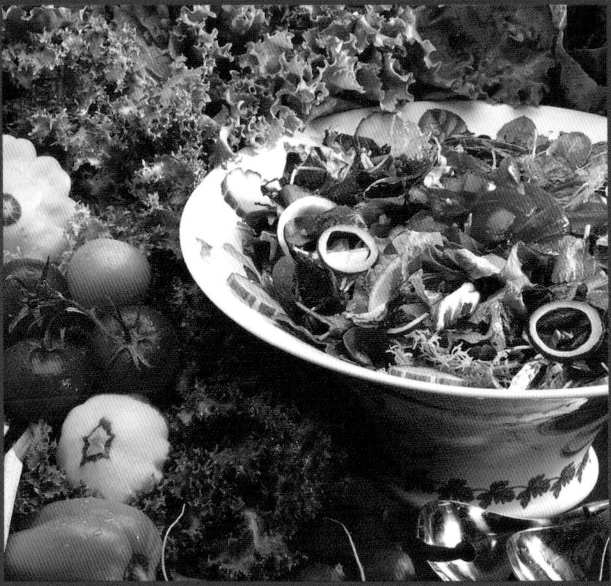

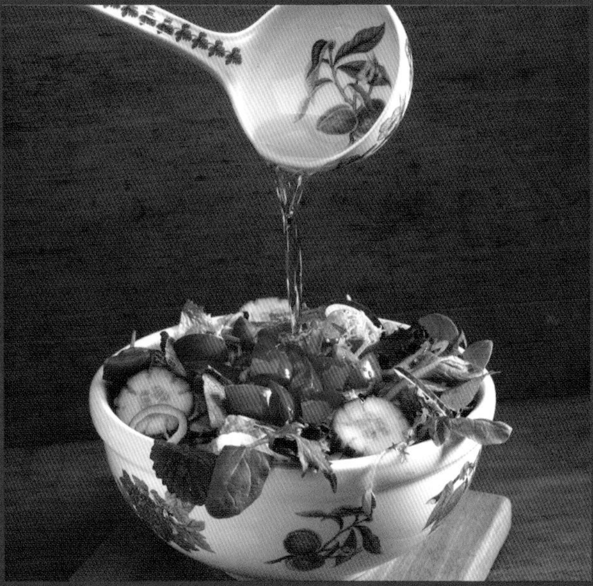

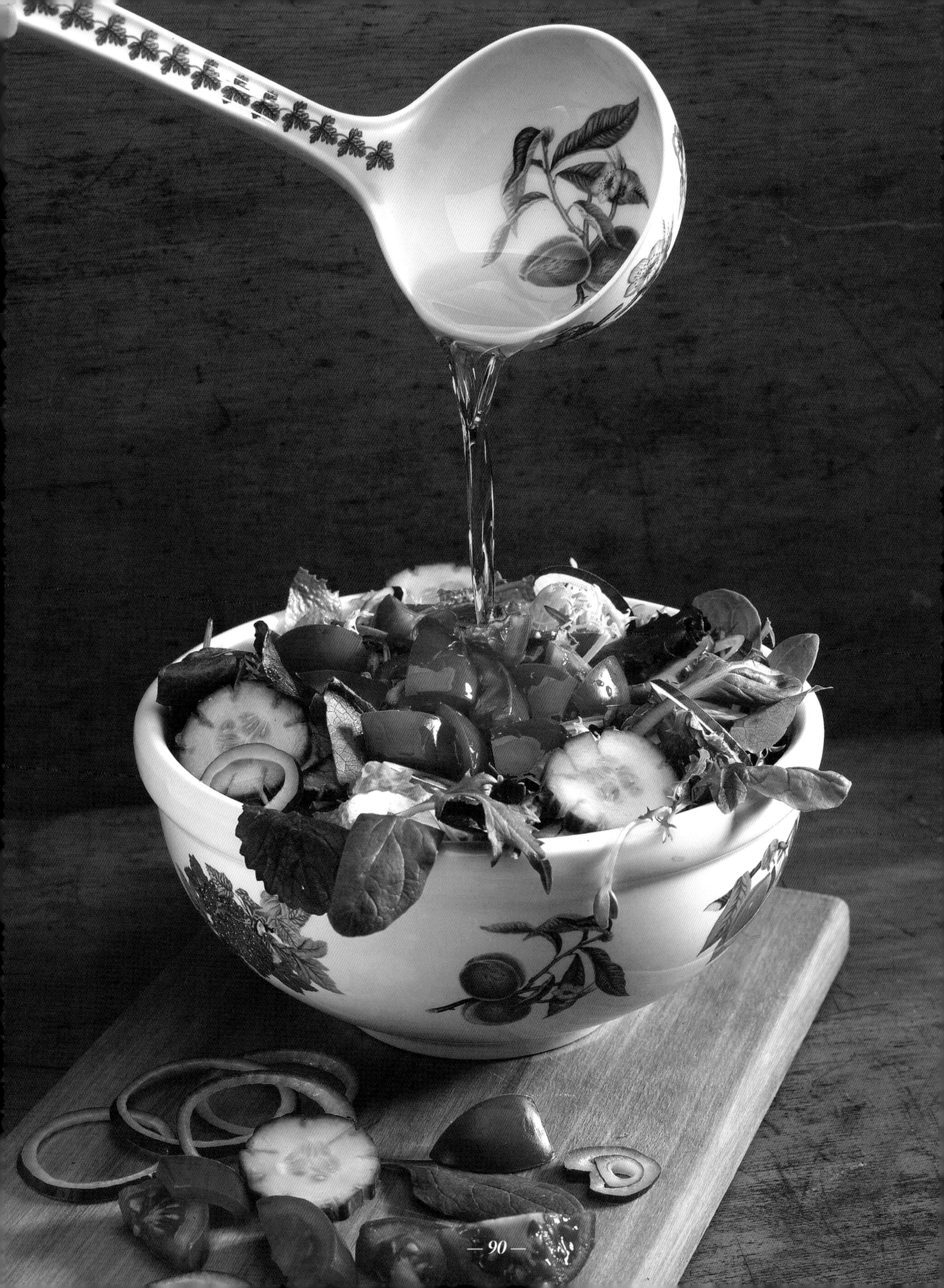

Chapter 7
The Art of the Salad

- What does 'Art of the Salad' mean?"
- How to build Whole Meals called Super Salads
- Our Super Salad Pyramid
- How to Overcome being Overwhelmed in the Kitchen,
- It's not Just poor Food Habits that are Making us Ill.
- The Secret Language of Nature.

Super Salads

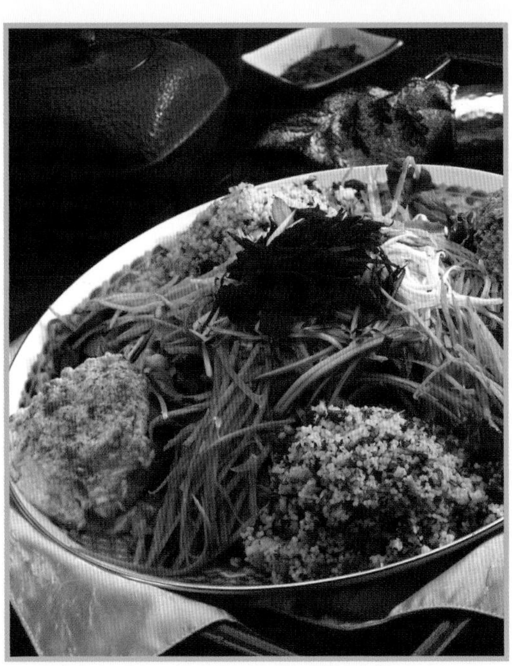

We've been conditioned to believe salads are a second thought. For the few who know the secrets I'm about to reveal, it's actually a rich world packed with wonderful, colorful varieties and combinations of vegetables. I have spent most of my adult life preparing, observing and studying how to make wonderful salads. Most of us don't understand that salads can be our best friend when it comes to meal preparation. They are incredibly easy to prepare, but, most of all, salads prepared our way are full of foods we would normally not eat, if we had to eat them separately. Plus, well prepared salads are full of colorful colored vegetables rich with phyto-chemicals, enzymes, antioxidants, vitamins and minerals. Mostly, they have a preponderance of fiber, something we all need in our diets. We like to call our salads, whole meal Super Salads, because truly they are an entire meal. That might freak some of you out a bit, because most people consider eating salads only the beginning of the meal. On the contrary, we establish that salads are the entire meal. Research shows over and over again that people who consume a high fiber diet have a very low rate of colon and rectal problems. It's no wonder. Our intestines are over 30 feet long! All vegetarian animals have the same kind of digestive structure. Their teeth, like human teeth are grinders. As humans, we do not have fangs to rip flesh from bones. We grind and chew our foods, the same as vegetarian animals. If our digestive tracts were three feet long, as most carnivore's are, then eating a preponderance of roughage would not be a healthy thing to do. John Robbins' book, Diet For a New America goes into depth on these and other relative issues. We highly recommend reading this book because not only is it a classic, it has information that will literally change your entire perspective on how we can better nourish ourselves on this planet.

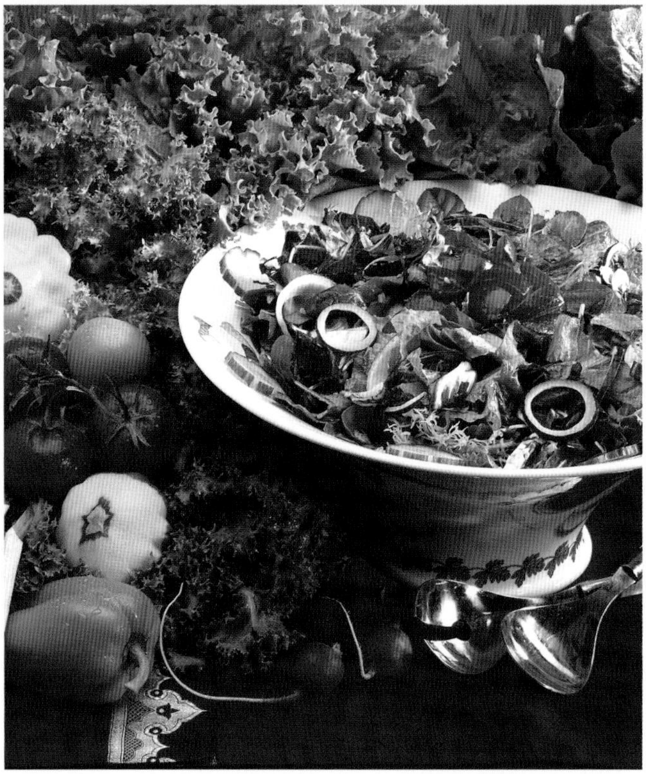

Salads Play a Large Role

What you will find, when you start eating more and more salads is that your energy will really start to accelerate, and your bowels will move with ease. There are so many attributes to eating salads, what Jay and I like to say, is please try it for at least two weeks. Then and only then will you realize this wonderful secret!

Salads are the CORE to our entire eating plan, and salad preparation, created as whole meals are incredibly easy to prepare; satisfying, and wonderfully liberating. Trust us: There is nothing boring about salads done our way.

When you learn to prepare these types of whole meal salads, you will find that prepared ahead of time, your entire dinner will not take you more than ten minutes to prepare. This does, however take some preparation ahead of time, but it's very minimal. We instruct you more in detail on how to do this on pages 95-97 Preparing these wonderful meals is very easy, and you will find also, that within the first two weeks of preparing salads our way, you will start to design them more for your tastes. You will soon become an expert. Is that great or what?

The Art of the Salad

What does "Art of the Salad" actually mean? By the time you finish this chapter, you will see and know there is more to preparing delicious, simple, yet satisfying meals than just through the mundane preparation of salad making. Furthermore, there is a lot more to being well than by just the foods we prepare in our homes, or even choices we make in restaurants. Let's start first with the most important aspect of learning an art:

Three Parts to Become an Artist:

1. Learning the basics
2. Committing to the entire process
3 Tuning into the unseen aspects of creating that puts our personal mark on it

1. Getting the Basics Down

I began to learn very quickly that simplicity was a ***must*** for us when it came to foods. I discovered this fact when, during the first week of our marriage, Jay came home from the grocery store and said, "Honey, I'm home." But what he didn't say was that he had fifty pounds of carrots on his back, waiting for me to cut, clean, and organize. "Hum," I thought. "I guess I'm going to have to become good at organizing and simplifying, because it will be a snowy day in the Amazon if I'm going to let him put all those fifty pounds of carrots in my little apartment refrigerator!" What I learned, back in 1981 about kitchen organization was a lot. There were many trials and tribulations along the way, but after about a year , I had it down pretty well. Being naturally organized was definitely not a forte of mine, so I realized that if I didn't make it fun and easy, life would be pretty unbearable for Jay *and* me!

I learned from Jay that to help keep our energy levels high, we needed to consume high quantities of green foods. This didn't scare me because I was raised by a mother who consumed a lot of green foods and juices; however, preparing whole meal salads was something I learned and experimented through trial and error.

Salads are Perfect Foods

Why? Because most people cannot digest heavy foods, including me, because of my digestive troubles. Interestingly, I noticed when I consumed 80 percent salads with 20 percent cooked grains or tofu, or beans, things went pretty well for me. I didn't get sleepy after I ate, (as I always did after I had eating a larger, more cooked meal). When I ate salads prepared this way, I was not bound up afterwards, and most importantly, my energy levels climbed very high. In addition to that, I felt satisfied after the meal, especially if I put nuts in the salads. That crunchy sound really went a long way with me.

What became so frustrating was that cookbooks in the '80'ss and most of the '90s just didn't discuss living foods whatsoever, nor did they discuss preparing whole meals via salad making at all.

Thus the concept of art of salad making came into being for me around 1988, two years after our two children were born. I started to experiment and study the basics of salad making. I knew salad making was simple in its practical form, but, as I said earlier, I needed to feel more satisfied when eating salads. This is when I started to add cooked grains, beans, and other goodies like sprouted seeds, nuts, and specialty foods such as Nori and tofu to our salads, and began creating

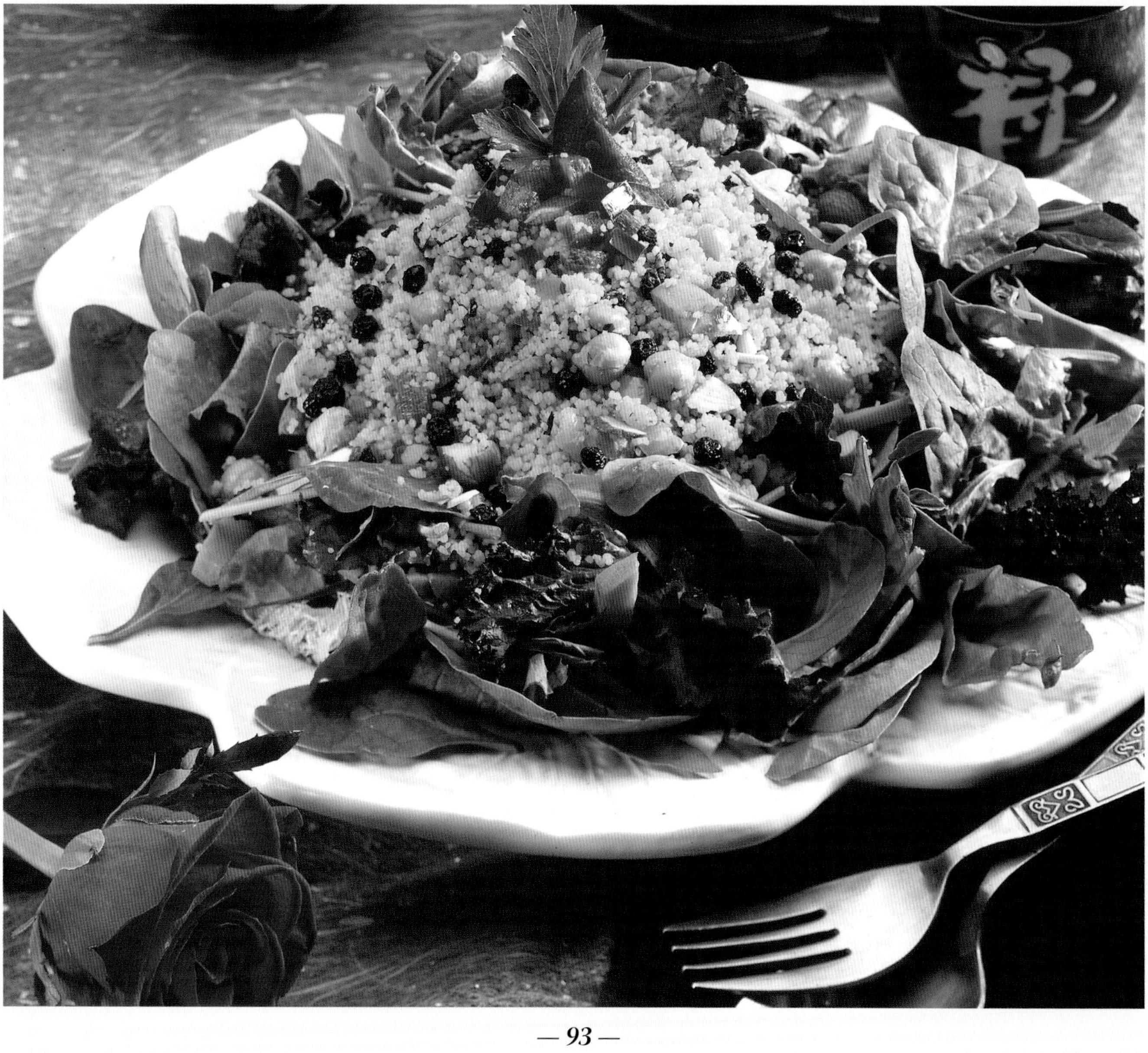

delicious salad dressings that went well with them. This is a very important fact when you are eating really good salads. I learned in studying Ayurveda that six tastes must accompany a meal for taste satisfaction and spiritual and emotional balance: astringent, pungent, sweet, bitter, sour, and salty. This is how my salads went from good to great.

Ayurveda (pronounced eye-yer-vay-duh) is the art of healthy living that enables you to create harmony in daily life by applying self- knowledge and self-care. The word, Ayurveda, is from the ancient Indian language, Sanskrit, and literally means "Knowledge of Life". Inherent in Ayurvedic principles is the concept that you are capable of taking charge of your own life and healing. Ayurveda may come from ancient texts, but these principles are just as applicable today in our society as they were when they were originally recorded in India thousands of years ago. Ayurvedic living occurs when you recognize your basic nature and live according to this true self.

Discovering Super Salads

I soon realized these salads became (what we like to call) Super Salads. Sometimes we would get creative, stuffing our salad into a tortilla, then pouring

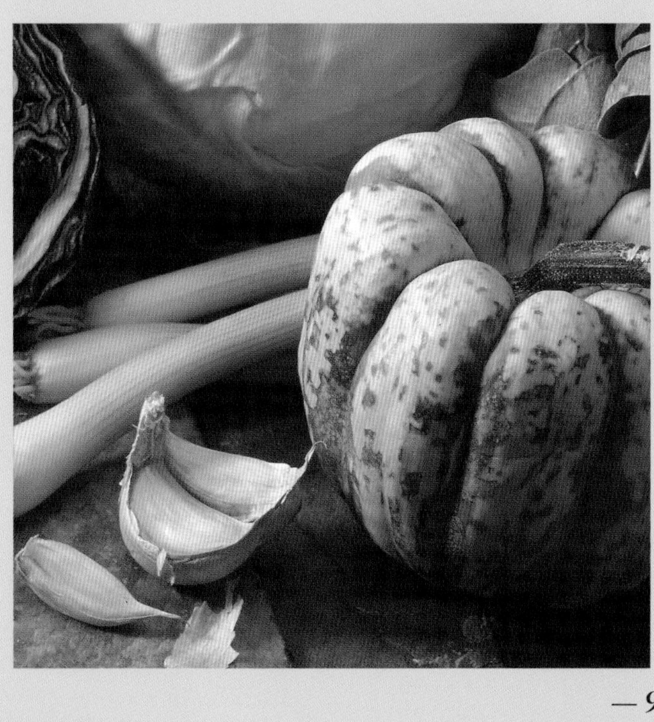

a wonderful dressing over the top. Our children liked eating their salads this way, too. It was simple, and it worked well even when we had guests over at the house, and prepared this way, it worked very well with our busy schedules. Once you learn our basics, you start making it your own by adding or subtracting certain seeds, nuts, and vegetables you like the best. For us, in particular, we love raisins in salads, which adds sweetness to all the other tastes we included into the salad.

Our Pyramid for Salad Making

You will find on the next page our salad pyramid, which shows all the different types of dried fruits, vegetables, seeds, nuts, grains, and sprouts you can create for your whole meal salads.

Just as an artist picks the colors and hues to paint onto his canvas to create a piece of art, thus the same is true for the salad—the bowl being the canvas and the foods being the colors and hues. Through time and experimentation, you will soon become an expert at making these wonderful one-dish wonders, and your body will love you for it. Trust me, within just five days, you will notice a significant difference in your energy levels and a more balanced bowel and nervous system.

However, if you suffer from colitis and/or diarrhea from eating greens, we suggest you read up on probiotics and enzyme therapy. Thousands of people have been helped tremendously by learning and integrating this wonderful practice of consuming enzymes and probiotics before or during meals. Most colitis victims have a very toxic colon, and an emotional life that is in turmoil, whereby the small and large intestine become tense and binds up. When this happens, our intestines because of this, evacuates the food immediately. This can be overcome, given the right nutrients and time.

Our Super Salad Pyramid

This pyramid flows from the bottom up, whereby the base of the salads will be salad greens. We show percentages to give you an idea of proportions. Remember to include all the six tastes for balance and satisfaction.

You can find more information about certain foods you can use in your super salads by looking on page 96-97 and for oils see pages 70-71 and more foods see pages 64-65.

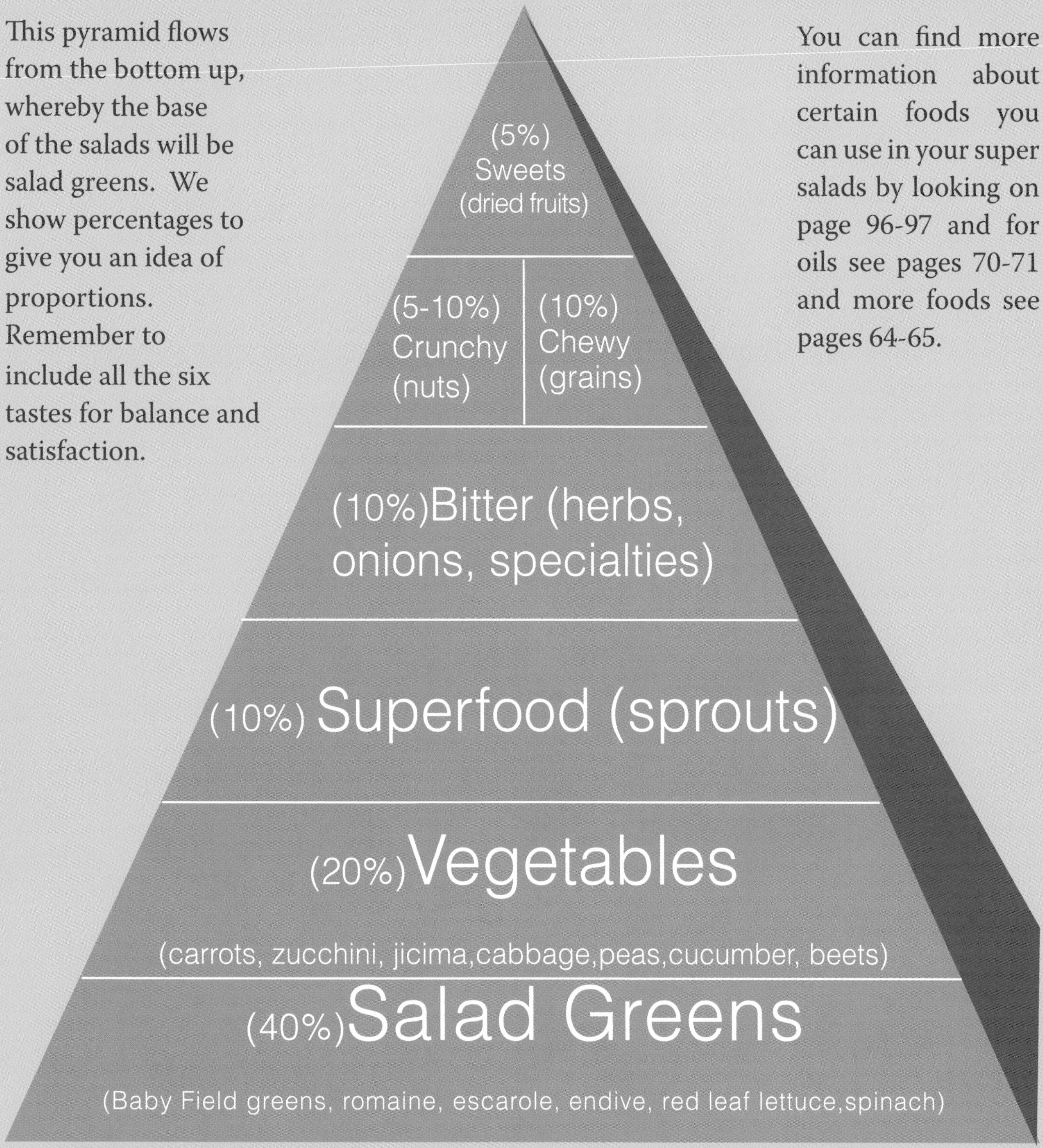

On page 106 you will find exactly what foods to use in your Salad Pyramid. In this Pyramid we are showing you the kinds of foods we use to create ourSuper Salads. This pyramid shows the base of the salad should be salad greens, evolving to the top, which is sweets, the least used ingredients. On page 96-97 you will many different kinds of possibilities mixed to your liking.

Super Salad Syn

GREENS for salads - Pick 3

Romaine
Red Leaf or regular Green Leaf
Baby Field greens or regular Field Greens
Cabbage, red or green*
Butter lettuce
Endive
Escarole
Arugula
Spinach (baby and/or regular)*

Vegetables for Salads (Pick 3)

Asparagus (steamed and sliced)
Bell Peppers (yellow, red, orange)
Cabbage, sliced thinly, green or red
Green Beans (steamed and/or cut in one inch pieces)
Jicima (julienned)
Beets* (julienned)
Fresh peas
Brussels sprouts* (sliced very thinly)
Cauliflower* (small flowerets)
Broccoli* (small flowerets)
Carrots* (julienned)
Napa cabbage (sliced thinly)
celery (chopped or diced)
Corn (cut off the cob)
Cucumber* (sliced in cubes)
Fennel (sliced thinly)
Jerusalem artichoke* (sliced thinly)
Peppers, red, yellow and orange*
Summer squash, green and yellow*
Zucchini*
Turnips
Cherry tomatoes
Plum, vine ripe and Roma tomatoes*
Edamame (cooked soy beans without the pods)

Superfoods: (pick 1)

Parsley
Sprouts
Alfalfa, Mung Bean, Adzuki, Lentil, Broccoli, Bean, Fenugreek, sunflower sprout

Sweets: (Pick 1)

Avocados
Raisins
shaved coconut (or flaked coconuts)
Dates
blueberries (small and regular)
Pomegranates
Currents
Dried cranberries, figs, apricots
Apples; any variety

amic Ingredients

Pears
Strawberries
Cherry Tomatoes
Roma tomatoes
Vine ripened tomatoes (all colors)
Special Heirloom tomatoes (all colors)

Crunchy (Pick 1)

Slivered almonds
Chopped filberts
Chopped walnuts
Chopped pecans
Macadamia nuts (chopped)
Peanuts (raw)
Sunflower seeds
Pumpkin seeds (tamari or regular)
Chopped or slivered nori sheets cut in strips

Chewy (Pick 1)

Short Grain Brown Rice
Cous - Cous (Israeli and regular)
Millet
Ancient Quinoa
Long Grain Brown Rice
Wild Rice
Pearl Barley
Lentils (brown or green)
Black Beans
Navy Beans
Potatoes -red, white or yellow
Tofu, firm, extra firm or medium firm (soft won't work)
Garbonzo Beans
Adzuki Beans
Black eyed Peas
Mung Beans (cooked)

Bitter/Astringent (Pick 1)

Fresh Basil
Fresh cilantro
Fresh Dill
Fresh Mint leaves
Leeks (sliced thinly)
Onions, white, yellow or red
Green Onions
Garlic
Organic Olives (pitted)
Radish
Radicchio
Shallots
Fresh Basil
Fresh Chives
Capers

A high percentage of digestive ailments have been helped tremendously in less than eight weeks when going on these types of programs.

There is so much to learn about probiotic health and superior digestion that it is well worth looking into. Jay has always said, "Death begins in the colon." Sounds drastic, but there's a lot of truth to this statement. Most of us feel very uncomfortable talking about bowel management, yet, ironically, it's the most important part to living health that we need to talk openly about. The most important thing we can do to be healthy is to build superior digestion, thus the reasons to bring it out into the open.

2. Commitment

Secondly, we want to commit to the belief we can change our lives for the better, especially to believe we can follow through with commitments. A commitment goes to our very core when it comes to changing a bad habit or addiction. This is why commitment is so crucial to any kind of change we want to make in our life.

> "When we learn the basics, when we learn to listen and integrate the unseen aspects of understanding an art, and when we mark it with our own flare, it's commitment to the entire process that weaves its permanent threads through each aspect of this wonderful new way of living and seeing life, literally from the *inside out.*"

Without commitment, we slip and slide, become unfocused, and give up. More devastating than that is that we tend to beat ourselves up emotionally for failing, damaging the already fragile foundation we once had.

So, you see, without committing, much of the teaching will fade. This is why when committing even if it's for ONE day, you will be proud of yourself when you finish. Then you can go from there and make it two days, etc. Even if you decide, to only commit for one week or one month, that's wonderful! Even if it's only two weeks, you can pat yourself on the back, knowing your life truly will change for the better after those two weeks. You will notice a difference, and even if you go back to your old way of living and eating, you will instinctively know how to get well again.

Being Addicted

Don't get me wrong, learning an art does not take thirty days. Integration may take up to a year to truly feel as if you have blossomed into a new being, and an artist at your own ability to make wonderful whole meal salads, but isn't it worth it? Better to try and fail than to not try at all. After all, I know a lot about failure. I am currently writing another book, which will be out in the next year, entitled My Kitchen Sanctuary—How foods that once imprisoned me have now liberated me. I failed for nine solid years with a food addiction called annorexia/bulemia, and then one day it all just changed. I was so exhausted and ill from the disease that I reached my lowest low. I had been married to Jay for close to two years, and was starting to change for the better, yet this addiction had been with me for so long, any good Jay contributed was washed away in a second when it came to trying to kill the evil I felt was controlling, dominating and directing my every food move.

One day, I woke up and told Jay that I really needed help, and I confessed my secret of being bulimic. Getting that off my shoulders and asking for help was a huge step. We didn't have any kind of insurance or money at the time, but he really helped me by putting me on a fast and getting me several colonics to help purify my system, helping to purify the old thoughts I held deep in my bowels. After ten days on this program and a lot of emotional purging on my part, I woke up after the following morning either on the tenth or twelfth day feeling as if I were free from something that held me as its prisoner for over nine years. In my next book, I will go into details, but for now, let me just say, transforming ourselves from food addictions takes a tremendous amount of courage, will, and grace from God. Only the fearless can pass through to the other side of our own dark shadow, but getting to the other side is worth it beyond words.

A New Day Begins

After I fasted for those twelve days or so, we did a lot more together to help, but this was a huge start. Even if you do not have an addiction as hard to overcome as mine, I'm sure most of us have addictions to food, alcohol or other related addictions that we have tried for a lifetime to overcome, yet we still seem to stay stuck in the same old song, playing over and over in our heads; "I'll never get thin, I'll never get well, this addiction has got me by the neck, I might as well just live this way. No matter what happens, I'll always seem to fail as failure mercilessly keeps pulling me under the water over and over again." Failing for nine solid years, every single day is depressing and overwhelming, yet I *did* it. You can too!

Believe me, when you start to eat green foods and especially vegetable juices, in a big way, you will start to break the addiction from the inside out, rather than from the outside only. You see, we must get control of that destructive voice inside of our heads that keeps us failing all the time!

Just like that little voice we just spoke about a few sentences ago. For some reason, vegetable juices, and eating greens daily actually gets to the core of our disorders and helps to eliminate the intense desire for simple carbohydrate foods such as pizza, sandwiches, ice creams and sugar foods, amongst others. Once we start to go back to these healing green foods, all the other negative habits get triggered

3. Learning to see the Unseen

There is one more suggestion I can give you: prayer. When we turn to the unseen, part of that is prayer. If you are not a spiritual person, then I would suggest seeing Nature as God. How could anyone deny this? Imagine: As you read this now, know that our earth is spinning, the sun is always rising somewhere on this planet, sweet delicious and colorful fruit is being born from trees as we speak, and life is being born and taken away as we circle this planet without any control from ourselves.

If you are a prayerful type person, ask God to help clean your body, heart and soul for a new type of eating and lifestyle. It may take time and especially effort on your part. This is how we really can change from the inside out. It's my personal belief that God answers us in the way in which he speaks: through Nature. It doesn't matter what religion we are, just pray to that higher force which inspires and guides us every day, even if we can't see it right now, the LOVE and support is always there.

Now we get into the part that is difficult to describe, because words sometimes fail, yet I will do my best, as the unseen is experiential, which is why words fail so frequently.

For me, the unseen became almost palpable when I began lighting candles and playing soothing music in 1990 when I started working in the kitchen more and more. It all started to come together for me then, after years of liberating myself from the food addictions that dominated my life until 1983. At this stage of my life, seven years after I had beaten the disease, I started to feel a spiritual force, or a special part of Mother Nature working through me as I started to create recipes for our future books. I started to realize that living foods had *life* in them. I started to realize spiritual and hidden aspects that related to the sun and trees, to the sun and berries, to the sun and vegetables, and especially towards the sun and my own body. I started to wonder about a lot of things. The more I wondered, the more answers I received.

As I started to learn to honor that new part of me, I truly felt I had beaten the deadly eating disorder that plagued my body and soul back in 1975-83. I started to see that my kitchen was becoming a sanctuary, rather than a place that held me captive. Learning this art is not just how we create our meals or what we put in them, rather it's integrating into ourselves this wonderful experience of Nature, seasonal eating, and most importantly learning to love ourselves and the sacredness of *life* throughout the process.

Turn Off the TV and Tune into Nature

Being a mother of two sons and running a huge business and home, I used to say I never had any time, but in truth I really did have time. I was spending most of my free time shopping, talking, socializing, going to the gym or just tuning out to de-stress. Once I started to slow down, spend more time alone in my kitchen, allowing these wonderful spiritual feelings to come through me, I completely changed. And it wasn't just the revelations about proper kitchen organization and healthy food eating habits. I had that down pretty good. It was something much deeper. I wanted to focus on those unseen factors that become the real factor to real change; change from the *inside* out. But most important was the spiritual connection I started to make between the incredibly beautiful foods Nature provided for us; colorful, beautiful, good for us, and perfectly backed right from the sun. Trust me, if there's anything you can take with you from this book, it's this concept: this spiritual *connection* belongs to everybody. Unfortunately, most of us as women have a very heavy plate when it comes to commitments and work, but please try to give yourself five hours per weekend to spend either gardening, taking long nature hikes, going to the beach, taking a class about plant life or just re-organizing your kitchen to start putting more LIFE into it. Most of us are always buying 'out' because it's easy, but in the long run, we all suffer. It disconnects us from our children and spouse and it teaches our children that nourishing ourselves is not found in the home, rather it's in restaurants. The bottom line is there's nobody in the kitchen, which can be taken metaphorically or literally. But it doesn't have to be that way.

Invite Your Children to Help

To change that old habit, try buying some flowers, light some candles, make your kitchen your sanctuary. If your kitchen intimidates you, I certainly understand. My kitchen was once my prison, now it's my liberator. Take it a step at a time. This is why 'ritualizing' it by starting to honor your kitchen is the first start. Next we need to start honoring the foods we chose to put into our kitchen. Next would be to add our children and/or spouse into the picture.

What I used to love to do, when our children were younger was to sometimes ask them to set the table for dinner with a theme, like color or style. It was really fun. One day we chose Mexican day, so we went shopping together, picked the foods out, then came home and chose a beautiful red table cloth with napkins colored

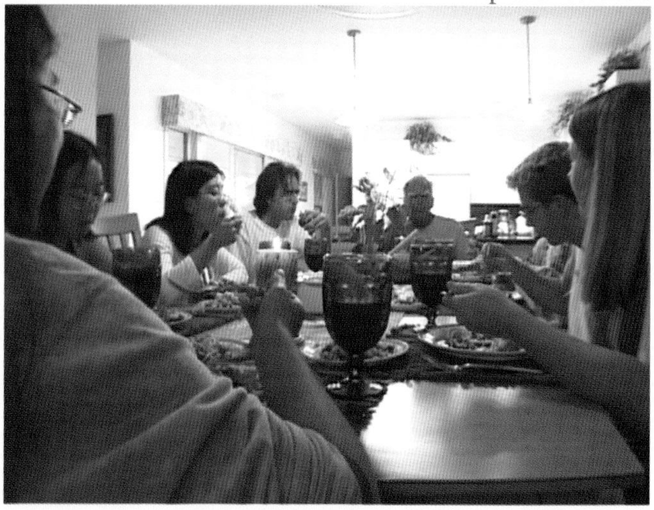

in every ray to set the table with. Our dishes didn't match, but we didn't care. Then we decided what we wanted for dinner that related to Mexican people and its culture. We ended up making wonderful vegetarian tacos and fresh lime juice margaritas (non-alcohol of course). What made it such a wonderful experience was that I had a chance to invite my children into the kitchen, create a wonderful meal with them, and they in turn, felt empowered and 'connected' to not just our experiences together, but to the whole process.

Breaking the Habit

We also need to disconnect ourselves from habitual and unconscious eating, because once we sit down to watch television, we lose ourselves watching TV and eating at the same time. Most of the time we can't even remember what we ate or how much we ate five minutes before. And for most of us who work for a living, this can become a chronic habit, especially if you live alone or have young children. Even if it's not TV, overeating is a chronic addiction that can be broken.

Here's a good way to break this habit

1. When you feel really hungry, drink some water right away before you get into the kitchen and start that unconscious nibbling. If you do not like water, add some emergen-C into the water. It will make it tastier. (Drink (8), 8-ounce glasses of water daily)

2. Do not turn on the TV, rather turn on the stereo and play some really relaxing music like Yanni or Enya, classical or subtle jazz music, while you're either preparing your meal and/or eating.

3. Light a candle and place it in the kitchen, and ask for patience and discipline so you may prepare and eat a healthy meal without feeling rushed. Rushing to eat is a trigger to overeating and poor food choices.

4. Set the table, then start to prepare what to eat.

5. If you have a grain already cooked and your greens already washed, it won't take longer than five minutes to prepare an entire meal.

Teaching children at a young age these kinds of kitchen rituals are a wonderful way to prepare them for kitchen habits they will use throughout their lives. (Please don't let them near the candles without supervision) After all, most of us Americans are over-stressed, overworked and incredibly overburdened. But this can change. We need to prioritize what's really important in our lives.

Think about it. Simplify your life. Take the stress out by cutting out all the extras that eat up all your free time. If you come home from work, and if you work with our system, you will have time to take your work clothes off and de-stress, before you start dinner. Don't go out at night, even if you children want to go somewhere. Allow one to two nights a week, rather than four or five.

Take your life 'off the hook'. Make your home your castle, and make your kitchen the place to relax and gather, rather than a place you avoid. Invest in yourself and your children, not the restaurants, nor the shopping centers. Once you start to detach yourself from this stressful type of living, you will start to enjoy all the free time you actually have.

I know what I'm talking about, because I have raised two children (as you most likely know are now 21 and 19). I built a company with Jay starting in 1981 that took all of our personal and work time, plus Jay was not home more than ten days per month, and we had two children during those times. We do know what it's like to raise children, have to work and then try to find personal time.

Simple Foods are Power Foods

Truthfully, simple foods *are* power foods. However, first let's make sure we are on the same wavelength here. Simple foods *are not* fast foods. Simple foods are foods that are naturally given to us by nature—fruits, nuts, seeds, berries, legumes, vegetables, and healing herbs. Interestingly, when we consume simple foods, our lifestyle begins to reflect the same.

Living a simple life is a divine right given to all, yet we, as a Nation lost it somehow. This is why spending a Friday night creating a wonderful dinner with our children is so powerful, yet is' so simple.

The disconnection must have started around the '50s when being number one as a Nation and as a personal goal suddenly took place as the mighty dollar reigned over family and simplicity. It really hit home for me because I was raised by a Norwegian grandmother whose entire life was one of simplicity. I witnessed for years as she prepared wonderful meals from her garden. Truthfully there was something magical about creating and preparing foods from that garden. That's how powerful simple foods and a simple life can be for you and your family.

You Have the Time!

I know what you're thinking again.... "I don't have time for that! After all, I'm overworked and underpaid, and especially under appreciated." Yes, it's true, but we let it happen. We've got to realize, *we* are the ones in power—that is, women are in power. We can decide how to delegate, how much time we are going to give ourselves for certain projects and how much time we are going to keep serving those who are unappreciative or appreciative of the work we so selflessly give to our families.

When we decide to eat a more simple diet and delegate some of the housework to our families, it indeed gets easier. But sometimes we like to endure the almost inherent 'martyr' in us that loves to say, "I'll do it, don't worry, just relax...." Sound like you? We can stop it, and it takes a little time, but trust me, with patience, understanding a little organization, your life will start to unwind, and you will have time to take that relaxing bath or sit out in the backyard and just listen to the birds if you feel like it.

As women, generally speaking, we are simple minded and incredibly loyal to those we love such as our children, family members and our husbands.

Martha Stewart is a good example of perfection. Perfection is not *real.* We love beauty, this is true, but we want to feel authentic and we want our lives to be authentic. Living by perfection principles ultimately creates failure, something we do not want you to experience.

With that in mind - Jay and I, for personal curiosities on our part, prepare a questionnaire every few years, whereby we ask women in our seminar audiences what their 'real' needs were in their lives. Here's what we found: (Not listed in order of importance)

1. **Save money and time in their kitchens**
2. **Lose weight**
3. **Prepare wholesome foods for themselves and their families--easily**
4. **Feel proficient and happy in their kitchens while they were working in their kitchens**
5. **Feel supported and helped by their spouseand/or family members in the kitchen**

Food Network Stars Let us Down

The Food Network would love to dupe you into believing you need to buy into the gourmet food regime. Is it entertaining? Yes. Is it empowering to us as women? Not sure. There are a few shows I sometimes watch where I get some applicable suggestions, but all in all, television food shows are not for me, and I become frustrated watching them entertain and create illusions rather than be of service to us women and mothers who have a lot more pressing problems than how to prepare a six-course, complicated dinner that evening. However, I am a true believer, that even if they don't target our direct needs, the information gathered can be a great help on several issues, such as product and food awareness. Think about our lives ten years ago, when the Food Network was a small channel, and few cable subscribers received their shows. Now, over 72 million Americans view these shows, bringing awareness about preparing foods at home, which we highly advocate. So with the fluff comes some great information I believe we can benefit from, although Jay and I would like to see some better shows on this network regarding healing foods and longevity issues.

Building the Salad Pyramid

On page 95, our Salad Pyramid helps you see how to construct a salad the way we design and construct our salads from home. These Super Salads are incredibly delicious, satisfying, and very filling. We highly recommend one large salad per day—either once in the afternoon for lunch, or at dinner time. We recommend eating your heaviest meal in the afternoon, and your evening meal the lightest. When the sun is at its peak in the afternoon is when our digestive juices are at their peak. This is when we should be eating our heaviest meal. This could be an old wives tale, but Jay and I started to use this principle about twenty years ago, and stick to it today, as it truly works. If you get hungry past 7 p.m., we recommend drinking a large cup of herbal tea, or eating a piece of fruit such as an apple or a pear, but nothing too sweet. Please do not eat any kind of crackers or potato chips, even if they're fat free - no matter how hungry you are. These foods can be dangerous in the evening time, when our digestive system and vital organs need time to rest and restore themselves before morning, thus the need only for foods that digest themselves without much effort.

Food Combining

Our Super Salad Pyramid shows you all the ways you can create your own whole meal salads. As a side note, I would like to say, combining proteins and starches can sometimes create gas and indigestion if you eat a large meal. If you keep your meals decent in size, it may not matter if you are combining protein and starches, depending on how sensitive your digestive tract is. On the contrary, juicing citrus with vegetables is truly a poor combination, which really does cause indigestion and gas. If you have other juicing books, you will see a preponderance of juice combination such as carrot/orange/cucumber or something like that. Many juicing books have recently been written by novices that really haven't studied deep enough to act as an authority. The only fruits you should combine with vegetables are apples. As Jay will tell you, apples have a very compatible alkaline/acid ratio with other vegetables.

Partners in the Kitchen: How We Do It

Jay and I have learned, because we are married and business partners, being partners in the kitchen is a must for us. Jay was reared with a different mentality, raised during the depression with a mother who didn't work, yet interestingly, he was open to balancing out our kitchen responsibilities without much convincing on my part. Perhaps this is because we teach foods and it was a natural evolution for us; however, I truly believe it's because he realizes how important it is to our children and those we teach that men *should* be partners in the kitchen. Why not? We as women work very hard, multi-tasking at all times. We need our husbands to be there for us, as a partner, on a daily basis. In turn, due to the fact Jay equals out the responsibilities, I'm emotionally motivated to make him a spectacular breakfast, (usually a wonderful living muesli and some stimulating tea.)

That's the best example of how we can be the most compatible partners in the kitchen. This should be our goal. We also have a rule. Twice a week, we both clean the refrigerator together. This is very important, because when we both clean together, we can see what we are not eating enough of, or vice versa.

Appreciation Goes a Long Way!

As a mother, I appreciate it when my family mirrors back to me the love and dedication I give to them, and it can manifest in mundane examples such as a family member cleaning up every night before they go to bed, to a more esoteric example like a beautiful card written to me telling me how much they appreciate the care I give to them. In our home we sometimes have three children living with us, all between the ages of nineteen and twenty-five. Because we have taught our children how to purchase natural foods, it's easy to ask them to go shopping for us, as it helps to alleviate added stress for either Jay or I when we prepare to make dinner. As your children grow older, try to teach them everything that you are learning about foods, especially fruits, vegetables and herbs. This will come in very handy for all of your family in the future. They will really appreciate what you have taught them as they grow older, especially if they bring home a friend and make them dinner with ease!

Here's other examples of how we work together at home:

1. Jay does our grocery shopping twice per week (on an average).

2. Our children take the groceries out of the car (if they're home) and take them out of the bags, then they store the bags in a drawer so we can return them to the store, which helps with the environment.

3. Jay and I wash the produce, clean it, and get it prepared for the rest of the week.

4. I organize the refrigerator so I know exactly what we have in the fridge, which helps me determine what we can creatively put together for that week.

5. I prepare the meals with our children if they are home.*

6. Jay cleans up in the kitchen before bedtime.

*Our children are nineteen and twenty-one, they instinctively know how to prepare meals without any assistance, and they know how to organize and operate a natural kitchen—something Jay and I wanted to make sure we taught them before they went off to college

Now that we have thoroughly discussed the Art of the Salad, let's get into the recipes!

Our Weekly Schedule

Monday

1. Shop for veggies/fruits/avocados/grains/nuts/tofu/seeds.
2. Drain water from Sunday's soaking (see sunday) of the sprouts you chose for this week.

Place in a dark area. rinse two times per day until ready, unless you have an automatic sprouter (GreenLife). Otherwise, use mason jars-they work great, but it takes more time than an automatic sprouter.

Tuesday

Soak nuts and or seeds for weekly meals before you go to bed. Clean out the refrigerator and clear out any foods that have gone bad. (make sure someone from your family helps.

Wed.

Rinse out nuts and/or seeds and and use until Saturday. Make sure to rinse your nuts every other day to make sure they stay fresh.

Thursday

Shop for Carrots and Greens.(Particularly for juicing.) Clean out the refrigerator.

Friday

Rinse first, and then soak grains overnight for Saturday cooking the next day.

Saturday

Farmer's Market shopping (in season foods)
Spend apprx. two hours preparing soup/grains (one soup and one or two grains for the week)
Wash all greens and store. Cut and clean carrots for juicing for the rest of the week.

Sunday

Soak seeds of your choice for sprouting for the rest of the week.

Remember - when you start to organize your natural foods lifestyle, you're actually building a living kitchen - an environment that cultivates living health, loving health and vital health for your family.

"Live Foods Bu

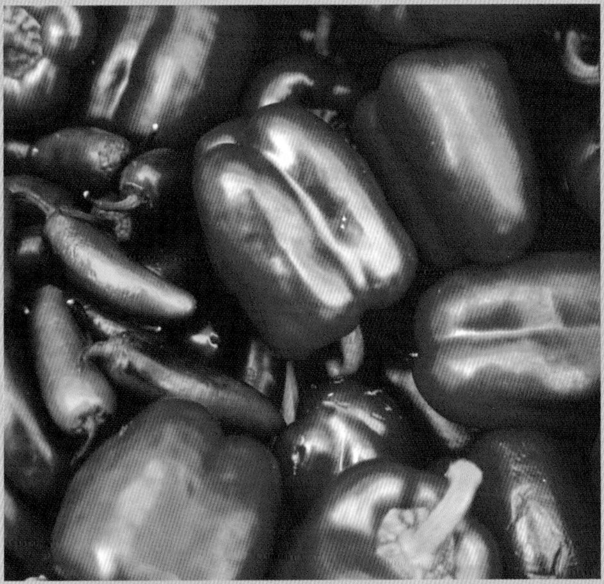

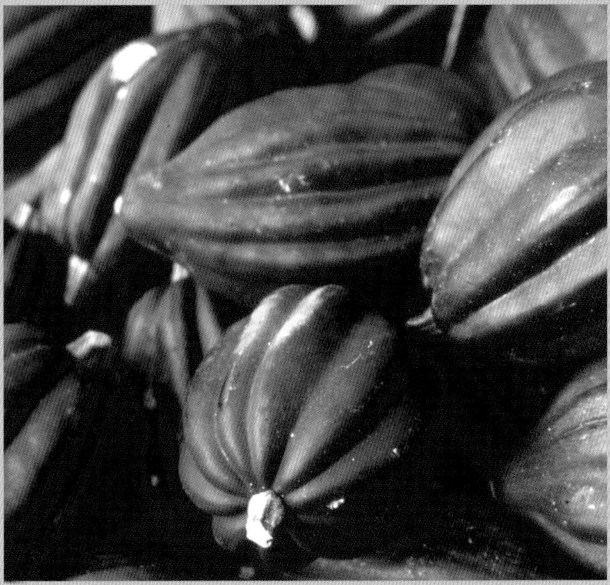

ld Live Bodies"

-Jay Kordich

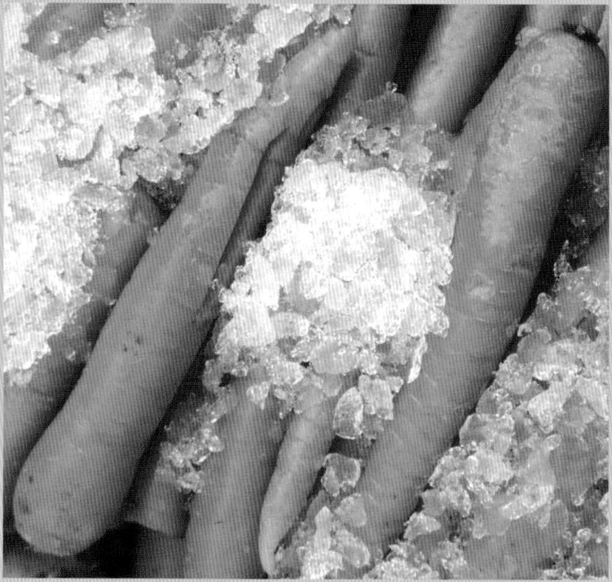

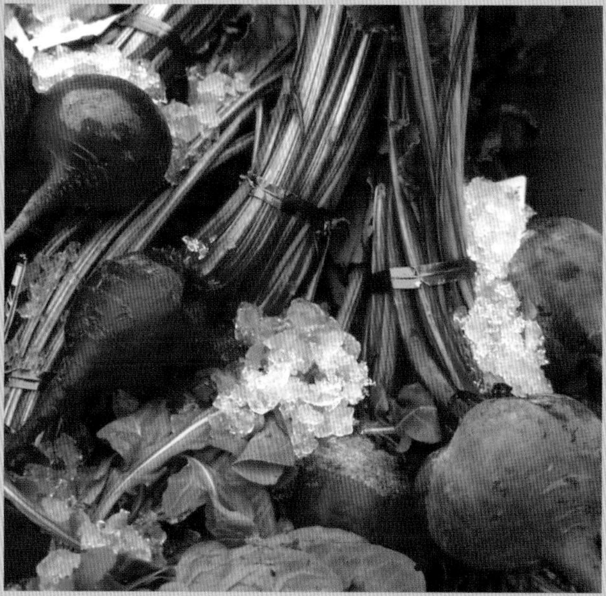

Menu

The Basics	112-121
Super~Salads	122-135
Living Soups	136-145
Pates & Dips	144-151
Dressings	152-163
Living Breakfasts	164-169
Living Breads & Crackers	170-173
Living Nut Milks	174-177
Energy Smoothies	178-185
Fresh Juices & Super Energy Juices	186-203
Acceptable Cooked Foods	204-217
Make your own	218-225

Chapter 8

Live Foods Live Bodies Recipes

In this section Jay and I share some of our recipes we have been creating and using for over 25 years. Our juicing recipes and smoothie recipes are the best you can find anywhere and are designed to help heal the body of degenerative diseases, including toxemia.

You will also find what we call **"THE BASICS."** The basics are designed to aid beginners in Living Foods to get started with foods such as Fruit and Vegetable Basic Salads In another section, we have Our whole meal Super Salads, which can be created from a green salad base, but to this we add either grains, soba noodles, potatoes or tofu specialties. If you are just getting started in natural foods, we suggest you start with the basics and within time, move your way towards our speciality salads and recipes.

Located on each page, we define which recipe is either 50, 75 or 100% living, or 100% cooked. #1 transition is 75-100% living, #2 transition is 50-75% living or # 3 transition is a 0%-50% living food recipe. This is more clearly defined when you decide to 'Take the Test; How Alive are You?', located on Page 33 in Chapter 3.

This will help you integrate and evolve into understanding how to incorporate more living foods into your diet on a daily basis without drastically changing your eating and lifestyle habits.

Our Super Salad Pyramid

On page 95 you will find how to build your own Super Salad Pyramid; the definitive and easiest and most creative way to construct wonderful whole food meals.

On all of our recipes we show our personal tips which will help you understand how to either make this recipe better by adding another recipe to it, or what juice you can add to it to make it more enzyme rich. As you most likely know, we want to make our recipes as 'alive' as possible.

Chapter 2 and Chapter 7

We suggest you read chapter 2, The Power of Living Foods, before you get into the recipe section to make sure you have all the ingredients you need to get started. We also recommend you read Chapter 7, Our Living Kitchen to learn about what living appliances you should start to collect so you may start to build a great support system in your kitchen.

Kitchen Magic - It can Happen

I would like to take some time to reiterate getting in and out of the kitchen in very little time when it comes to preparing mealtime. (We discuss this in Chapter 6, pages 85-86) Preparing beforehand is the key to fast natural food preparation. On our program you will spend an average of about 2 hours per Saturday (or whatever day you are off) preparing cooked soups of your choice, washing and storing greens, vegetables and fruits. You will also be spending some time preparing a grain for the next five days. When you have grains, greens, veggies, soups and fruits organized and prepared ahead of time, you have got it made for the rest of the week. Now you can go out to eat on Friday or Saturday evening without feeling guilty because you have prepared healthy, vital and energetic meals earlier that week! Imagine all the money you also saved preparing a several quarts of soup for a few dollars, instead of one cup for $3.50 or so. It's incredible how much money manufacturers make on selling one small cup of soup for anywhere between $1.50-$5.00! And the prices are sky high with frozen foods, canned beans, packaged cereals as well.

Interestingly, most people think eating a healthy diet is complicated and intimidating, yet almost all of our ingredients are very easy to find and to make. There are only a few that are challenging to find, which would be the young baby coconuts. If you live in the mid-west and your regular grocery store does not have them, you will find them very easily in Asian Grocery stores. (Bring your children, teenagers or grandchildren with you). We highly recommend you treat yourself to a day like this! It's so interesting to see how other cultures eat, and you will indeed expand your horizons as a result. Further, if you do not want to venture out to do something different, ask your grocer-he can special order the products.

. Baby coconuts are one of the most perfect mineral and enzyme rich foods we can consume, including having some of the most perfectly balanced fats for a healthy heart and vascular system. Please try to find the book, The Coconut Oil Miracle, by Brian Fife, N.D. You will be amazed at the wonders of pure coconuts and their oils. Just be very sure only to purchase unheated coconut oils for your salads. Our suggestion is to purchase your coconut oils from Eatraw.com. Nama Shoyu, which is easy because it's actually Tamari, better known as Soy Sauce. However Soy Sauce is usually full of ingredients that are not natural, and Tamari is a wonderful substitute because it's wheat free containing natural ingredients. Interestingly, Nama Shoyu is soy sauce, yet it's not been cooked or heated so it's a fermented product, containing healthy living enzymes. We prefer Nama Shoyu for this fact, yet if you cannot find it in your grocer, we highly recommend Tamari for those of you who do not want to search. You will find this in our web site and resource section of our book, but it's worth mentioning again. Jay and I highly recommend you use 100% pure, extra virgin organic olive oil, or 100% organic and uncooked coconut oil, or 100% organic and uncooked macadamia nut oils for consumption.

Obviously, the refrigerated efa oils (essential fatty acid) omega 3,6 and 9 oils are recommended. Udo Erasmus' oils are highly recommended. We read his book many years ago (when conventional medical doctors were still touting margarine as being a better choice) back in the early 1990's called: Fats and Oils. It is the definitive book on fats and oils.

So you see, from our home to yours comes a plethora of information to help you and your family make the right choices. Jay and I do not financially participate with any of the companies we recommend to you, and for good reason. We do not want to be persuaded by anyone or any company to promote their products.

We hope you enjoy your new energy and vitality through this new lifestyle. We ask that you love yourself and your family and especially share this wealth of knowledge. The more we change our eating habits, the more the food manufacturers and retail food outlets will change too. I can remember back in 1964, when I was only nine years old, my family could only go to Chinese restaurants or Seventh Day Adventists cafeterias to get vegetarian foods. Now there are more and more Juice Bars (thanks to Jay!) and vegetarian restaurant choices. Imagine if we all just keep this up? We will create a healthier future. Jay and I are not sure if you realize just how unhealthy we are as a Nation. Ironically we are the richest nation in the world, yet the most unhealthy. We are almost at the bottom of the charts in health scores for the entire world We attribute this to too much stress, demanding jobs, and poor quality foods. Too many animal products and foods such as: pre-packaged sugared foods, canned foods, and fast food restaurants all attribute to this.

Eat at home we say. Simplify your life and start creating a rich life for yourself and your family right in your own kitchen and your own home!

Our Natural Food Pyramid

One serving equals about 1/2 cup, so when we say weekly for sweets, oils and breads, that means up to 1/2 cup per week. The exception is honey. Only up to one half cup is recommended per week. We should be consuming at least 5 pounds of salads per week. That would include all the ingredients such as rice, beans, tofu and other additions put into your super salads.

Grains (see pages 64-65)
Beans: (see pages 64-65)
Nuts: (see pages 64-65)
Sprouts: (see pages 64-65)
Breads: (see page 171)
Greens: (see pages 64-65)
Fruits: (see pages 64-65)
Veggies: (see pages 64-65)
Oils: (see pages 64-65)
Sweets: (see pages 64-65)
Juices: (see pages 20-21 and 187-203)
Tofu: (see pages 64-65)

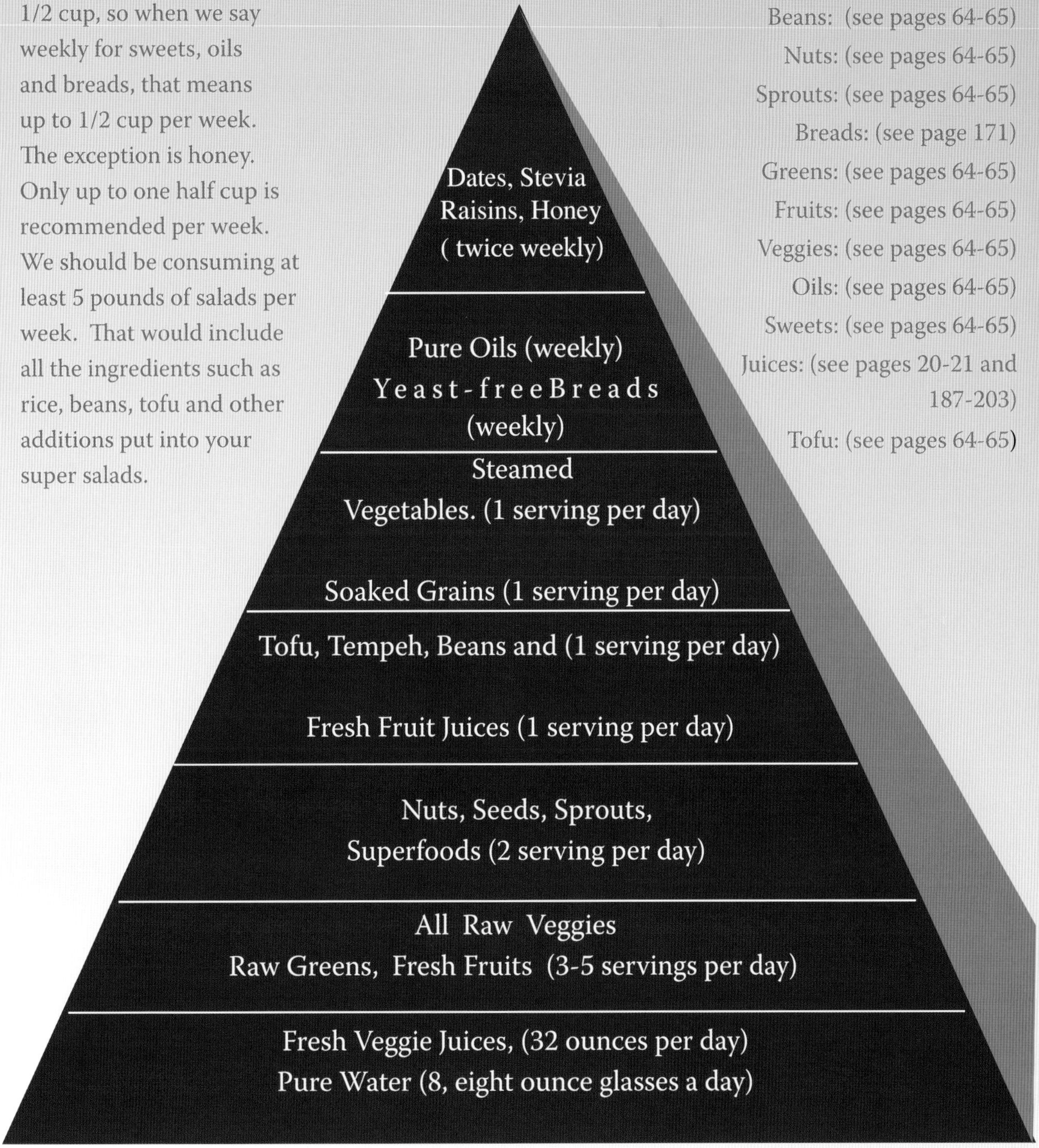

This is our Natural Food Pyramid we created to illustrate living food choices for our daily diets. The most foods you should be eating will start from the bottom with it flowing to the top where we eat smaller portions. As you can see we offer a wide variety of fruits, nuts, seeds, vegetables, herbs and legumes, some of which are cooked.

Our "Basic" Recipes

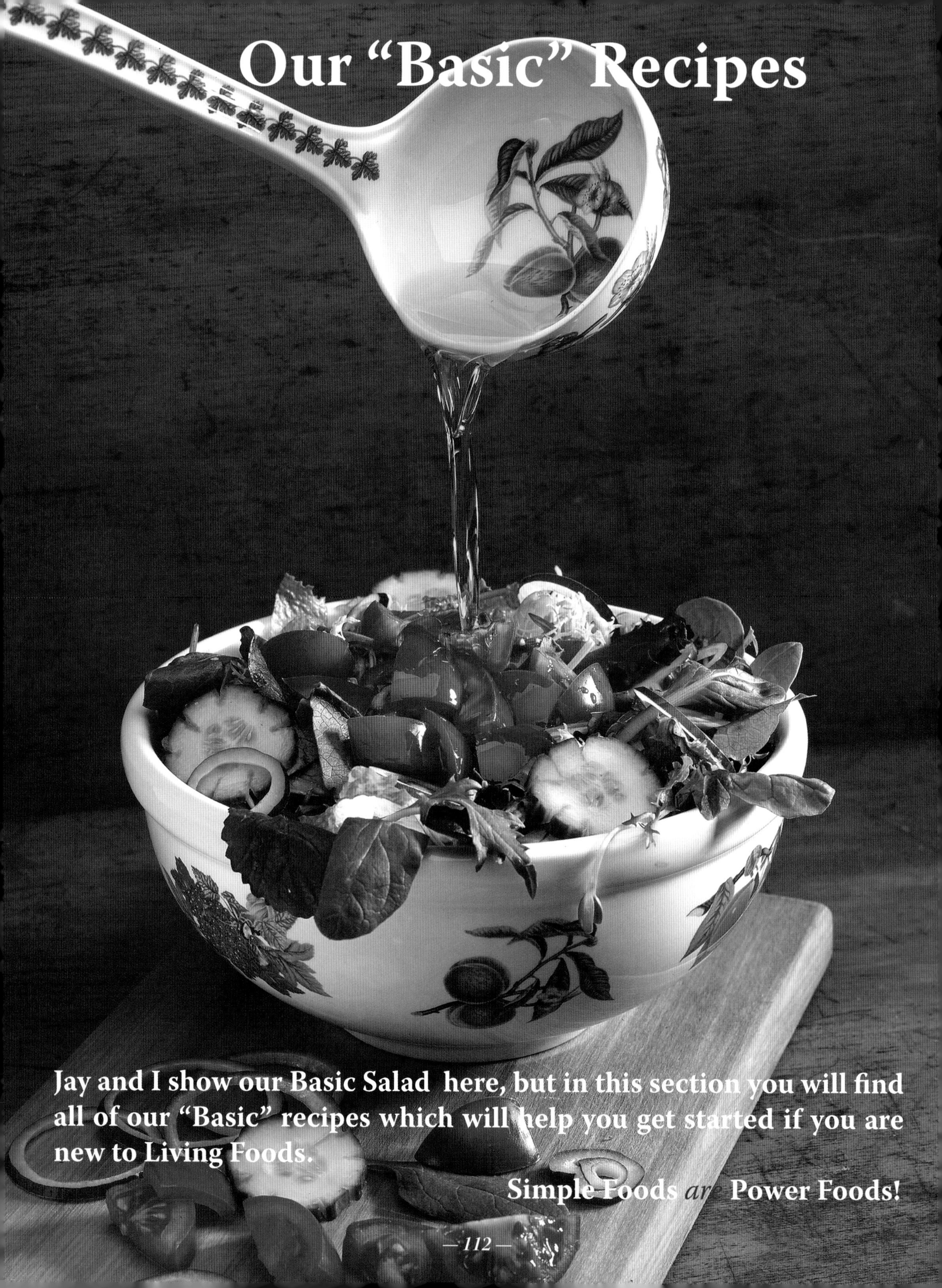

Jay and I show our Basic Salad here, but in this section you will find all of our "Basic" recipes which will help you get started if you are new to Living Foods.

Simple Foods *are* Power Foods!

Prep Time: 5m | Serving: 2 | 100% Living

1. Our Basic Salad

Ingredients:

1	Large head of Romaine Lettuce, chopped
1/2 cup	Red onion, sliced in rounds or slivers
2	Vine ripened Tomatoes
1	Peeled Cucumber
1 cup	Organic Spinach (regular or baby)

Directions:

Wash and spin romaine lettuce and spinach until dry, and then cut into bite size pieces. Chop onion into slices or rings, depending on how you like it. Chop tomatoes into one inch pieces, and peel cucumber and slice into rounds.

Linda's Tips:

This is a great salad for consuming with cooked meals. It's simple and easy to make, and it adds a lot of living food into your cooked meal to help make it more alive.

1a. Our Basic Dressing

1/2 cup	Extra virgin organic olive oil
1 tbsp.	Nama shoyu or Tamari

Directions:

Whisk olive oil and tamari slowly together until the ingredients have jelled together. This is a great dressing wen you're in a hurry.

Linda's Tips:

If you do not want to use Tamari in this recipe then you can substitute it for 4 tbsp. of either fresh lemon or lime juice and one clove garlic.

❀Prep Time: 20min ❀Serving: 4 ❀75% Living

2 Basic Rice Salad and Basic Dressing

Salad Ingredients:

3 cups	Carrots, shredded
6	Green onions, minced
2/3 cup	Fresh parsley, minced
4 cups	Cooked Brown Rice (short grain)
8	Large Romaine lettuce leaves, chopped (for garnish)
2	Large Tomatoes, cut in wedges, (for garnish)
3/4 cup	Black olives, pitted (for garnish)

Ingredients for Salad Dressing

1/4 cup	Fresh Lemon Juice
2 tbsp.	Tamari
1 tbsp.	Dill weed, crushed and fresh
1/2 tsp.	Sea salt
1/4 tsp.	Black pepper (or to taste)
2 tbsp.	Extra virgin olive oil

Directions:

In a mixing bowl, add lemon juice and stir in Tamari, dill weed, salt and pepper. Slowly whisk in oil and beat until well blended. Set aside. In a serving bowl, combine carrots, green onions, and parsley. Add rice while it is still hot and mix well. Toss with the prepared dressing and serve garnished with the romaine lettuce leaves, tomato wedges and black olives.

Linda's Tips:

Choose one of our Digestive Aid recipe on page 20-21 with this salad. You can use a variety of different fresh herbs to add more living foods into this recipe and also julienned raw veggies such as zucchini, bell peppers and/or steamed broccoli or cauliflower. A good addition in this respect would be recipe #8.

Prep Time:20m | Serving: 4 | 60-75% Living

3. Our Basic Soba Noodle Salad

Salad Ingredients:

1 pound	Green soba noodles, cooked according to pkg. directions
1/2 cups	Broccoli florets
1/2 cup	Green zucchini, julienned
1/2 cup	Yellow zucchini, julienned
1/2	Green beans, steamed and cut in half
1 head	Romaine lettuce or baby field greens
1 cup	Napa cabbage, sliced thinly
1/2 cup	Red bell pepper, diced
1	Small tomato, chopped
1 cup	Black olives, pitted and chopped
3/4 cup	Red onion, cut in rings

Dressing:

1 cup	Olive oil
1/3 cup	Fresh basil,chopped
1/3 cup	Fresh lemon juice
3 cloves	Garlic
2 tbsp.	Pine nuts

Seasalt and Pepper to taste (or cayenne instead of pepper)

Directions:

In a blender, combine basil, lemon juice and garlic and pine nuts. Slowly add oil while mixture is processing, and blend until smooth. Meanwhile, in a steamer, steam broccoli and green beans until crisp-tender. In a serving bowl, place romaine leaves on the bottom, toss and combine remaining salad ingredients and mix well. Toss with dressing and serve..

Linda's Tips:

Soba Noodles are easy to find. In any Asian market you can ask for them or you can find them at a health food grocery store. They are also known as Buckwheat Noodles. This is a wonderful recipe if you like heavier salads. This is an Italian/Asian/American fusion of a great salad! Digestive Juice Aid recipe # 12 on page 21 goes really well with this salad. This dressing lasts up to

Prep Time:10m Serving: 2 100% Living

4.John's Basic Living Spaghetti

Ingredients:

2	Green zucchini
2	Yellow zucchini
6	Medium sized vine ripened tomatoes
2	Large cloves of garlic
1/2 cup	Fresh organic basil
1/2 cup	Olive oil
1 tsp.	Sea salt or to taste
1/2 tsp.	Black pepper or to taste

Pure water for consistency desired.

Directions:

Pulse in a blender the tomatoes, oil, basil, garlic, salt and pepper with as much water needed to achieve acquired consistency for your sauce. We use about 1/2 cup.

John likes it really chunky, but you may prefer it more smooth. If so, blend at high speed for approximately 30 seconds. Grate Zucchini julienned style, or use a spirilizer for special effects to make it look more like real spaghetti.

Linda's Tips:

You can add pine nuts into the recipe. Just sprinkle the nuts over the top of the spaghetti. This is a great summer dish. We recommend our Basic Salad with this recipe located on page 113. and our Basic Flax Crackers on page 172, recipe #54.

Prep Time:20m | Serving: 4 | 100% Living

5 Basic Living Pie

Crust:

1 1/2 cup	Sunflower seeds (raw)
8	Fresh medjool dates
1/2 cup	Organic Raisins

Put into food processor and blend for approximately 3 minutes, or until mixture starts to bunch up whereby oil is starting to loosen up from the sunflower seeds. Now it's good and pliable for making into a pie crust.

Filling for Fall/Wintertime:
Bananas (thinly sliced)
Pears (thinly sliced)
Apples (shredded)

Filling for Spring/Summertime:
Strawberries (thinly sliced)
Peaches/Nectarines(thinly sliced)
Boysenberries/blackberries (whole)

Topping:

(Use young Baby Coconut water and all it's meat can be used for topping year round when combined with Banana) Papaya, coconut and/or mango for spring/summer or Banana/Blueberries and/or Coconut for wintertime. Sometimes we add the following spices to our toppings: 1/2 tsp. of Organic cinnamon, nutmeg, or cloves. Add 1/2 tsp. liquid vanilla Then blend all together.

Puree papaya and coconut and/or mango and coconut to a thick but not too thick puree. Same goes for Fall/Wintertime fruit choices. Pour over top of the pie , then sprinkle dried (unsweetened) coconut flakes over the top. Chill for one hour before serving

Linda's Tips:

Our Basic Pies are incredible. There is no sugar added, strictly fruit, nuts, seeds, loaded with heart healthy fats, proteins and perfectly digestible fruits. Whatever the season, we recommend you use the fruits in season, but use no more than three different fruits in each pie. Use strawberries, mangos or papayas for Spring/Summertime and, Bananas/Coconut meat for Fall/Wintertime's topping.

Prep Time:10m | Serving: 2 | 100% living

6. Basic Fruit Salad and Dressing
(Spring and Summer)

Basic Fruit Salad

2	Medium Nectarines, cored and cut into 1 inch slices
2	Medium Pippin apples, seeded and thinly sliced
2	Ripe Peaches, peeled, pitted and sliced
1	Ripe Banana, peeled and sliced
1 cup	Strawberries, sliced
1/2 cup	Walnuts, chopped
1/4 cup	Coconut, shredded (organic and packaged without sugar is ok)

Lemon for garnish

Dressing: (same for recipe #7, on page 119)

Directions

Crack coconut (see recipe #62, page 182 for directions.) Put water and coconut pulp into blender with ginger, macadamia nuts and vanilla. Blend until it becomes cream. In a serving bowl, combine salad ingredients to the dressing and toss. Remember to use a bit of lemon juice over the top to prevent browning of the apples and other fruits, if you are going to store the salad before you put the dressing on. This salad will last, under refrigeration for 12 hours.

Linda's Tips:

Sometimes if we are eating this salad for breakfast, and we have time, we will blend fresh orange juice with organic fresh macadamia nuts, add some honey, vanilla and nutmeg and blend until we reach a good consistency for a topping over the salad. It's a great addition and full of protein and fats - perfect living recipe to get you started for the day!

Prep Time:10m | Serving: 2 | 100% Living

7. Basic Fruit Salad and Dressing
(Fall and Wintertime)

Basic Fruit Salad

2 Medium bartlet pears, seeded and cut into one inch slices
2 Medium Pippin apples, seeded and thinly sliced
1 Medium banana
1/3 cup Chopped walnuts (raw)
1/3 cup Sunflower seeds (raw)
1/3 cup Flax seeds (for garnish)

Dressing

1 Baby coconut including water
1 inch fresh ginger root (peeled)
1/2 cup macadamia nuts
Dash of Vanilla and honey if desired

Directions:

Crack coconut (see recipe #62,page 182 for directions.) Put water and coconut pulp into blender with ginger, macadamia nuts and vanilla. Blend until it becomes cream. In a serving bowl, combine salad ingredients to the dressing and toss. Remember to use a bit of lemon juice over the top to prevent browning of the apples and other fruits, if you are going to store the salad before you put the dressing on. This salad will last, under refrigeration for 12 hours.

Linda's Tips

When you decide to use this recipe, make sure the pears are ripe. However just as an fyi; when you juice pears, they should be firm, so they juice better. Fall time is wonderful for a variety of different types of pears. This makes for a great breakfast start.

Prep Time: 5m | Serving: 2 | 100% Living

8. Our Basic Shredded Veggie Salad

Ingredients:

Julienne the following:
1 Cup Jicima
1 Cup Zucchini, green
1 cup Carrots
1 Cup Beets

Veggie Salad Dressing:

1/2 cup Olive oil
2 tbsp. Fresh Tarragon
1 tbsp. Apple cider vinegar
1 clove Garlic

Seasalt and black pepper to taste
(or cayenne)

Directions:

Blend apple cider vinegar, garlic and fresh tarragon in blender, then add the olive oil slowly. Will last up to seven days in refrigerator. Mix all shredded veggies into a bowl and mix with our Basic Veggie dressing above.

Linda's Tips:

This is a wonderful recipe for additions to other recipes such as our basic salad recipe #1 on page 113. Also it's great to use this recipe inside some of our wraps located on page 175 recipe #56.

✽Prep Time:5m ✽Serving:2 ✽60-75% Living

9. Our Basic Oatmeal

Ingredients:

4 cups pure water
1 teaspoon sea salt
2 cups steel cut oats

Additions:

1/2 cup raisins
1/2 cup nuts, chopped
1/2 cup dates, chopped
1/2 cup fresh fruit
1/2 cup apple, grated
1/2 cup pear, grated
1/2 teaspoon cinnamon
1/4 teaspoon nutmeg
Dash of Organic Flax seeds for garnish

Directions:

In a large saucepan, boil the water. Add oats and salt, stirring frequently. When oatmeal has thickened, remove from heat and add any of the additions listed above. Cover and let stand for 5 minutes. Place in individual bowls and serve with flax seeds, honey, and rice milk over the top. In the summertime, soak the oats for an hour instead of cooking them, and you have a muesli styled, uncooked oatmeal.

Linda's Tips:

This is a wonderful recipe for additions to other recipes such as our basic salad recipe #1 on page 113. Also it's great to use this recipe inside some our wrap's located on page 175 recipe #56..

Our Super Salads

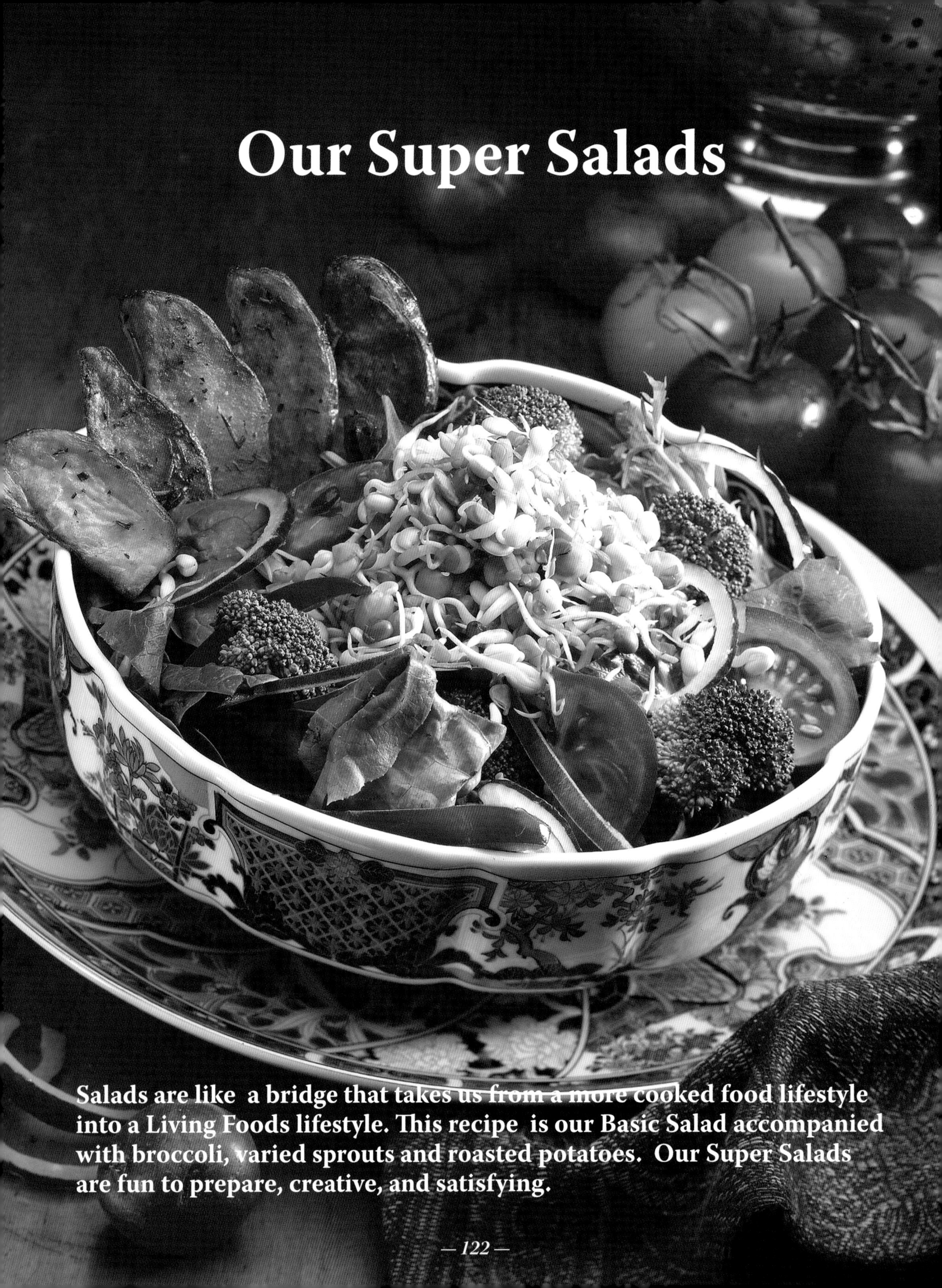

Salads are like a bridge that takes us from a more cooked food lifestyle into a Living Foods lifestyle. This recipe is our Basic Salad accompanied with broccoli, varied sprouts and roasted potatoes. Our Super Salads are fun to prepare, creative, and satisfying.

Prep Time:10m | Serving: 4 | 100% Living

10. Seaweed Spinach Salad

Ingredients:

3	Nori sheets (seaweed sheets 10x10 inches)
3 cups	Baby Field Greens
1/2 cup	Spinach
1/2 cup	Sunflower seeds
1/2 cup	Pumpkin seeds

Julienned or grated:

1/2 cup	Carrots
1/2 cup	Zucchini
1/2	Red bell pepper

Directions:

Place all ingredients together into a large bowl, except for the Nori sheets.

Under a gas fire (BE CAREFUL) lightly toast nori until is shrivels up (should only take a few seconds).

Use your hands to crumple up the nori sheets into the salad, whereby they look as if they have been crushed into 1 inch pieces. Next proceed to adding the dressing.

Dressing:

Our Basic Dressing # 1a on page 113. Variation: Add the following ingredients to the basic dressing: 2 cloves garlic, pinch cayenne pepper, 1 tsp. sesame oil and 1 tsp. fresh Tarragon.

Blend together in blender.

Linda's Tips:

This is a great recipe for women. Research shows nutrients found in Seaweed are great for our hormones. I like to add a cup of cooked Brown Rice to this salad to make it a Super Salad.

Prep Time:10m | Serving: 4 | 75-80% Living

11. Jay's Favorite Whopper Salad

Ingredients:

5 cups	Organic Baby field greens
1 cup	Organic Baby Spinach
1/2 cup	Walnuts, chopped
1/2 cup	Organic raisins
1/2 cup	Raw cashews, chopped
1 cup	Grated carrots
1 cup	Grated yellow or green zucchini
1 large	Vine ripened tomato, chopped
1 cup	Cooked garbonzo beans
1/2 cup	Green onions, chopped
4	Organic spinach tortillas (for wrapping)

Directions:

Place greens into a large bowl. Add rest of ingredients Toss – then add dressing when you are ready to serve. Heat the tortillas until warm and wrap all the ingredients inside, if you choose to eat your salad this way.

Linda's Tips:

Jay loves to eat this salad with a heavy veggie juice drink such as #7 Digestive Juice Aid, on page 21. We add a lot of dressing into this type of salad burrito, because the dryness of the tortilla is transformed by the generous application for the dressing. We recommend dressing #44, on page 160.

Prep Time: 10m | Serving: 4 | 100% Living

12. Healthy Protein Salad

Ingredients:

2 cups	Romaine lettuce
2 cups	Baby Organic Spinach
1/2 cup	Raw cashews
1	Grated carrot (or julienned)
1/2 cup	Chopped walnuts
1/2 cup	Minced parsley
1/2 cup	Raw sunflower seeds
1/2 cup	Bean sprouts
1 cup	Lentil sprouts (or any kind of other sprouts)
2	Small avocados, chopped (or 1 large Haas avocado)
1	Large vine ripened tomato, chopped
1	Small green onion, diced for garnish on top

Directions:

1)Toss all ingredients together except avocados
2)Top with sesame Tahini Dressing # 46 on page 162
3)Garnish with slices of avocados and chopped tomatoes on top.

Linda's Tips:

This is a whole meal in itself, loaded with protein. This salad goes well with Digestive Juice Aid # 2 on page 20.

Prep Time:15m | Serving: 4 | 75% Living

13. Mid-Eastern Salad

Ingredients

1 1/2 cups	Bulgur, uncooked
2 cups	Boiling water
1 to 1 1/2 cups	Dark, plump organic raisins
21/2 cup	Fresh mint, diced
1/2 cup	Minced fresh parsley
1/2 cup	Chopped green onions
2	Cucumbers, peeled and chopped
2 to 3	Fresh vine ripened tomatoes, chopped/de-seeded
1/3 cup	Extra virgin organic olive oil
1/2 cup	Chopped olives
3/4 cup	Fresh lemon juice
3 garlic	Cloves, minced

Seasalt and Red pepper to taste

Directions:

Pour boiling water over the bulghur in a large bowl. Cover loosely and let stand for an hour. Drain well in a colander and place in large bowl/container. Add other ingredients and toss well to combine. Add olive oil, minced garlic and lemon juice at the end. Chill a few hours before serving. Better the next day, as all the flavors have had time to blend in.

Linda's Tips:

I love putting this salad over any basic salad as a total meal, or stuffed inside my tacos recipe #90 on page 212 or inside a large green cabbage leaf. (My personal best is doing it the cabbage leaf way-try it - you will love it!) Thirsty? Try Digestive Juice Aid #11 on page 21.

Prep Time: 5-10m | Serving: 4 | 75% Living

14. Mock Tuna Salad

Ingredients:

1/2 cup	Diced celery
1/2 cup	Organic relish (store bought)
1/2 cup	Unrefined sesame oil
1/2 tsp.	Sea salt
2 tsp.	Nama shoyu or tamari
1/3 cup	Nutritional yeast
1 tsp.	Kelp powder
1/8 tsp.	Black pepper
1/8 tsp.	Cayenne pepper
1/2 pound	Cooked garbonzo beans

Directions:

Soak garbonzo beans overnight – then cook for approximately 2 hours via pressure cooker. When they are easy to mash, they are ready. Add the rest of the ingredients into the blender and blend coarsely until desired consistency is achieved.

Linda's Tips:

Love this recipe on sandwiches, on top of salads with little protein and fat, somewhat like our basic salad #1, on page 113, and this recipe is great with our flax seed cracker recipe # 54 on page 172.

Prep Time 15m: Serving: 4 100% Living

15. New York Cabbage Salad

Ingredients:

1 1/2 cup	Diced red and green cabbage
1	Medium apple, diced
1/2 cup	Organic Almonds, (soaked) and sliced
1/2 cup	Organic Raisins
1/3 cup	Pomegranate seeds (or substitute for dried cranberries)
1/2 cup	Fresh Cilantro, diced
1	Head Romaine Lettuce, diced

Dressing:

1/3 cup	Apple cider vinegar
1 tbsp.	Honey
1/2 cup	Pomegranates (or dried cranberries)
1/2 cup	Macadamia nut oil
2 tbsp.	Fresh Lime juice

Seas Salt and cayenne pepper to taste

Directions:

Put all ingredients for salad into a bowl. Place salad over a bed or red large leafs for color. Blend dressing with whisk and slowly add oil until desired consistency has been reach.

Linda's Tips:

This is a beautiful salad, incorporating a lot of different tastes and gorgeous colors. No need for a digestive aid tonic, as this is a totally 100% living meal. But, since you are using cabbage, we suggest recipe # 12 on page 21 if you so desire!

✽ Prep Time: 10m ✽Serving: 2-4 ✽ 75% Living

16. Better than Egg Salad

Ingredients

1 lb.	Organic extra firm tofu
1	Clove garlic
2	Large celery stalks, diced
1/2 can	Diced black olives
1/2	Diced yellow onion
1/3 cup	Nayonnaise (or any egg free mayonnaise)
3 tsps.	Organic Dijon mustard

Sea salt and Pepper to taste, adding just a pinch of cayenne pepper

Directions:

1.) Crumble tofu with your hands into a mixing bowl
2.) Add remaining ingredients and mix together

Linda's Tips:

If your extra firm tofu is very wet, we suggest you squeeze out all the water and pat with a paper towel. It's crucial your tofu is dry for a successful recipe. Spread it on Rye Crisp or flaxseed crackers, #54, page 172. I also love it on top of a simple green salad (our basic salad #1 and 1a for the dressing on page 113) .

Prep Time:10m | Serving2 | 60-75% Living

17. Super Salad Wrap

Ingredients:

2 cups	Romaine lettuce, shredded
2 cups	Alfalfa sprouts
1 cup	Lentil or other sprouts-your choice
1 cup	Carrots, julienned
1	Medium cucumber, peeled & sliced
2	Medium tomatoes
1 1/2 cup	Black beans
6	Green onions, chopped
3	Ripe avocado, peeled, pitted, diced
1/2 cup	Our Favorite Salsa (#33, page 148)
4	Spinach tortillas (warmed)

Directions:

Very easy to prepare. Start with tortilla. Make sure tortilla is warm enough to wrap without tearing. Spread tortilla with layer of beans, followed by avocados, carrots, cucumber, lettuce, sprouts and then salsa.

Linda's Tips:

Our kids loved this recipe when they were little. This recipe goes well with Digestive juice recipe # 33 on page 148. Sometimes I like my burritos a little more wet than normal, so I put an extra dollop of a pate or dressing we may have in the refrigerator before completely wrapping it up. Pate # 36, Homemade Humus goes well with this salad.

Prep Time: 15m | Serving: 4-6 | 60-75% Living

18. Asian Salad

Ingredients:

4 cups	Cooked short grain organic brown rice
6	Minced scallions
1/2 cup	Raw cashews
1/2 cup	Chopped dates
1/2 cup (each)	Fresh minced parsley and cilantro
2 tbsps	Chopped fresh mint
1 tbsp	Crushed, fresh dill weed
1	Sliced Tomato (for garnish)

Dressing:

3 tbsps	Bragg's or Nama Shoyu
1/4 cup	Organic Olive oil
1/4 tsp	Freshly grounded black pepper

Directions:

In a large mixing bowl, add hot rice mixture first. Then add all the other dry ingredients together. Next add dressing. Mix and serve. Garnish with chopped tomatoes, and if you are really hungry, add an organic, sliced Haas Avocado on top as well.

Linda's Tips:

If you are really hungry and want to make this a heavier meal, add along with the tomatoes, sliced Haas Organic Avocados on top. Our Digestive Juice recipe # 8, page 21 is great with this meal.

Prep Time:10m | Serving: 4 | 60-75 % Living

19. Simple Walnut Rice Salad

Ingredients:

2 cups	Cooked short grain brown rice
1 cup	Grated carrots
1 cup	Chopped walnuts
1 cup	Any sprouts (lentil, alfalfa, mung bean, adzuki)
1	Chopped green scallion

Special Dressing for Walnut/Rice Salad:

1 tbsp	Sesame tahini
2 tbsp	Bragg's
4	Large leaf fresh basil
2	Cloves garlic
2 tbsp	Sesame oil (unrefined)
1 tbsp	Fresh lemon juice

Directions:

Blend dressing and toss with salad ingredients

Linda's Tips:

This is a great addition to any 100% living salad, such as recipe #1, Our Basic Salad listed on page 113. You can toss it together, or place on top of the salad. Use the dressing listed above if you do combine our basic salad with this walnut rice salad. Digestive juice #3 on page 113 is great with this salad.

Prep Time 15m: | Serving: 2-4 | 60-75 % Living

20. Millet Basil Salad

Ingredients:

1 cup	Cooked Millet
1/3 cup	Basil
1 cup	Chopped Romaine lettuce
1 cup	Baby Spinach
1/2 cup	Chopped red tomatoes
1/4 cup	Diced white onions
2 tbsp	Diced green onion
1 cup	Carrot, julienned
1/2 cup	Diced cucumber
1/2 cup	Cilantro or parsley

Directions:

On the stove top take two cups pure water and one cup millet and cook approximately 30 minutes, or until the millet has absorbed all the water, whereby the millet looks done.

In a separate bowl, place all the ingredients inside except for the onions and cilantro and/or parsley and tomatoes.
When the millet is done, place on top of the salad and mix together with the salad. Finish with the tomatoes, onions, cilantro and/or parsley for the top.

Linda's Tips:

This is a wonderful salad where you can substitute any grain and make different variations this way. I love to add Pumpkin seeds to this recipe to give a more texturized flavor, and we like to use salad dressing #43, on page 159. Thirsty? Try Digestive Juice Aid #10, on page 21

Prep Time: 10m | Serving: 2 | 60-75 % Living

21. South of the Border Salad

Ingredients:

1 cup	Red leaf lettuce, chopped
1/2 cup	chopped cilantro
1 cup	Romaine lettuce, chopped
4	Chopped medium tomatoes
2	Diced avocados
2 tbsp	Lemon juice
1/4	Diced yellow onion
10 ounces	Cooked beans of your choice

(Our choice: pinto, navy, white, or garbanzo beans)

Directions:

Wrap the above ingredients inside of large green cabbage leaves. Add dressing #42 on page 158 onto the top of this recipe after you place into cabbage leaf or tortilla.

Linda's Tips:

I prefer this recipe adding cooked garbonzo beans. Or in a more traditional manner, you may wrap this salad into a tortilla. We would recommend a spinach tortilla. We suggest Digestive Juice Aid #1, page 20.

Prep Time:10m | Serving: 2 | 100% Living

22. Jay's Favorite Beet-Apple Salad

Ingredients:

1/2 cup	Chopped organic (raw) walnuts
2	Golden or green apples, cored and diced
4 cups	Red leaf lettuce or romaine lettuces
1	Medium sized beet, julienned

Dressing:

1/3 cup	Organic Walnut oil
3 tbsp.	Fresh lemon
1 tsp.	Organic mustard
1 clove	Garlic

Salt and red, or black pepper to taste

Directions:

Prepare salad and put all dressing ingredients into the blender except for the oil. Slowly add the oil as it is blending until it looks completely blended.

Linda's Tips:

Jay really likes this salad in the fall, and will add slices of ripe pears to this salad. Eating raw beets is especially great for the liver, and when combined with apples, it helps your liver even more, as this is a great combination for good liver/gallbladder function. Need more liver stimulation and rejuvenation? Try The Liver Stimulator #79 on page 200.

Our Living Soups

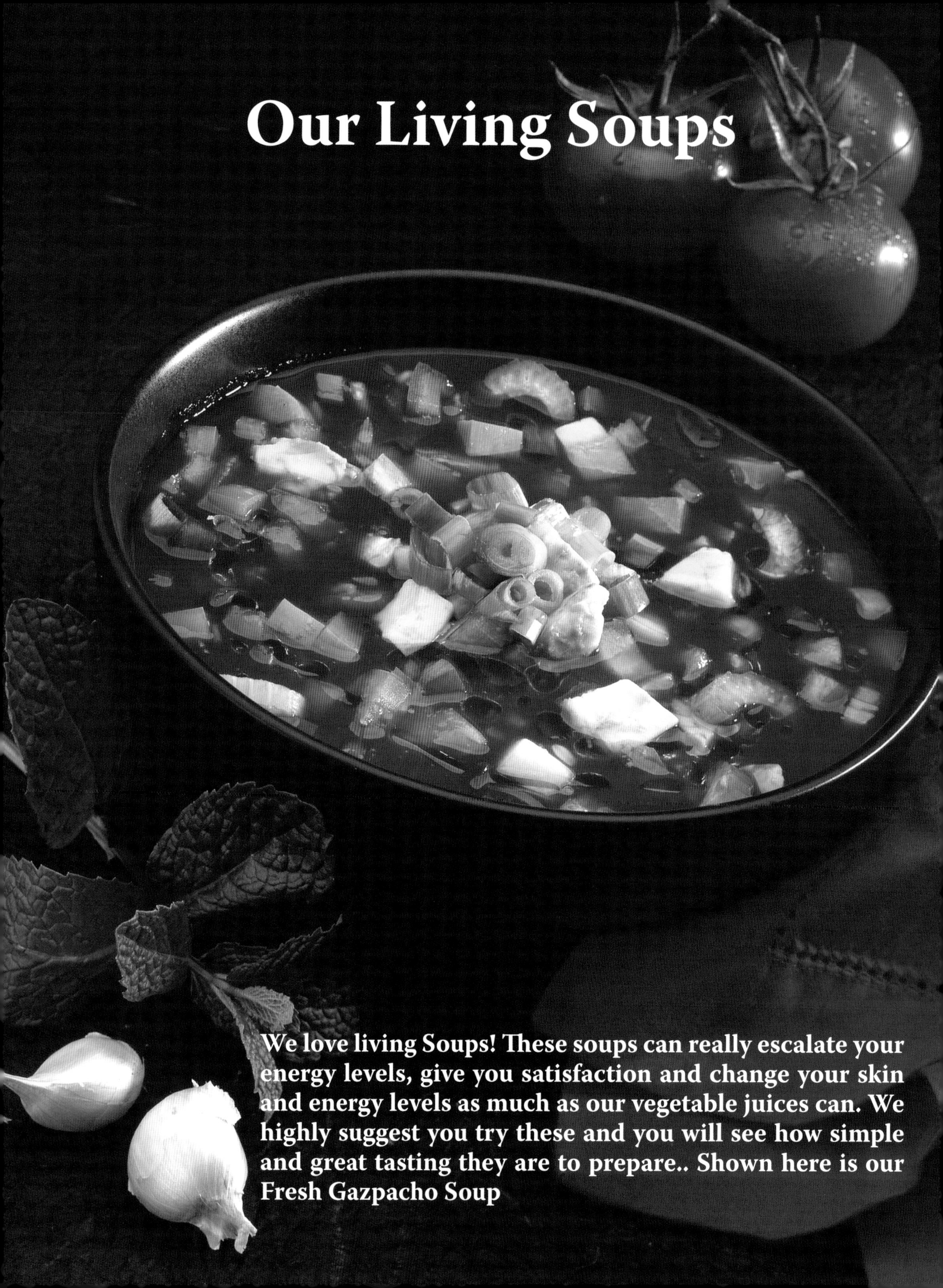

We love living Soups! These soups can really escalate your energy levels, give you satisfaction and change your skin and energy levels as much as our vegetable juices can. We highly suggest you try these and you will see how simple and great tasting they are to prepare.. Shown here is our Fresh Gazpacho Soup

✽Prep Time: 10m ✽Serving:4 ✽ 100% Living

23. Our Fresh Gazpacho

Ingredients

4 cups	Fresh tomato juice (juice apprx. 6 tomatoes)
3 cups	Tomato, diced
1-1/2 cups	Cucumber, peeled and diced
1/2 cup	Green bell pepper, diced
1/2 cup	Fresh cilantro, chopped
2	Stalks celery, diced
2	Ripe avocados, peeled, pitted, and diced
5	Cloves garlic, minced
2 tbsp	Olive oil
1 tbsp	Fresh lemon juice
1/2 cup	Green onions, chopped (for garnish)

Directions:

In a large mixing bowl, combine all the ingredients and mix well. In a blender, add half of the mixture and blend until smooth. Pour blended ingredients into mixing bowl and mix well. Cover and refrigerate for 3 to 6 hours. Serve cold and garnished with chopped green onions.

Linda's Tips:

This soup is energizing because it's 100% living. It's a great soup to go with any whole meal salad which is semi-cooked such as recipe #19, Simple Walnut Rice Salad. It also goes great with our recipe #88 or 90, Tofu Tacos and/or Vegetarian Tacos.

Prep Time: 5m | Serving: 2 | 100% Living

24. Ruby Ambrosia Living Soup

Ingredients:

1/2	Organic Beet
2 tbsp.	Fresh basil
2 tbsp.	Raw tahini
1 clove	Garlic
1/2 cup	Fresh lime juice
1 inch	Fresh ginger, peeled
1/2	Cucumber peeled
1/3_	Yellow onion (medium)
2	Medium sized tomatoes, vine ripened
1/3 tsp.	Celery salt

Sea Salt and Pepper to taste

Directions:

In Blender: Put all ingredients except for cucumber. Pulse and/or blend until desired consistency. We add the cucumbers last because sometimes if we blend everything, it gets too creamy, you can blend in the cucumbers in the last minute and only blend for 20 or 30 seconds, to give a more thick soup.

Linda's Tips:

This is a wonderful soup for cleansing, and especially for the liver. I love to eat our Flax Seed Cracker recipe #54, on page 172 with this soup to give it a crispy taste.

✽Prep Time: 5m ✽Serving2 ✽ 100% Living

25. Luscious Living Soup

Ingredients:

1 cup	Fresh spinach
1 cup	Purified water
2	Tomatoes, vine ripened
2	Cloves garlic
2 tbsp.	Sesami tahini
1 tsp.	White miso
1 tsp.	Salt
1 tsp.	Black pepper

Directions:

Blend all ingredients together until desired consistency is achieved

Linda's Tips:

This is my favorite soup. I only blend for about thirty seconds, because we personally like this soup a bit chunky. This soup is so easy to make – it literally takes two minutes to prepare. Try preparing our Super Salad Wrap on page 130 to go with this recipe.

Prep Time: 5m | Serving:2 | 80% Living

26. Jay's Magic Living Soup

Ingredients:

12	Carrots (for 2 cups carrot juice)
2 inch	Fresh Ginger Root, peeled
1/2	Fresh Lime, juiced
1 lb.	Soft organic tofu*
3	Cloves garlic
2 tbsp.	Sesame tahini
2 tbsp.	Tamari or Nama Shoyu
1/2 tsp.	Black Pepper
1	Medium green zucchini, julienned
2	Stalks Celery, chopped
2 tbsp.	Fresh Parsley minced
1/2 cup	Fresh Cilantro, minced

Directions:

In a juicer, juice carrrots with ginger and lime. In a blender, combine prepared juice with tofu, garlic, sesame tahini, celery, Tamari or Nama Shoyu, and black pepper. Blend until smooth. Pour mixture into serving bowl and add zucchini, parsley and cilantro. Stir until well blender. Cover and refrigerate 1-2 hours before serving.

Linda's Tip:

Why is this a magic soup? Because every time I make it, it disappears Kidding aside, this is a great soup, Try our basic salad # 1 on page 113 to go with this soup. Can be made without tofu, just substitute white miso (2tbsps.) for the tofu.

✽ Prep Time:5m ✽ Serving: 4 ✽ 100% Living

27. Jay's Quick Energy Soup

Ingredients:

8	Medium sized carrots
1/2	Small beet
1	Avocado, Haas style
1 tsp.	Cumin
1/8 tsp.	Cayenne or 1 inch square of fresh jalapeno pepper

Seasalt and Pepper to taste
Garnish: chopped organic tomatoes, cilantro and green onions on top.

Directions:

Super easy soup – just put all ingredients into your blender, blend until it reaches consistency you like. (We like it a bit thick). Garnish with chopped tomatoes and cilantro on top. Try eating our soba noodle salad # 3 on page 115 with this recipe.

Linda's Tip:

This is a fantastic soup in the summertime. Just remember to only use Haas avocados – they are the best avocados we have used for years. The other avocados are not as oily or rich in taste.

Prep Time: 10m | Serving: 2 | 100% Living

28. Cleansing Living Soup

Ingredients:

1	Large green zucchini
1	Medium red bell pepper
1 cup	Parsley
1 cup	Cilantro
2 tbsp.	Tamari or nama shoyu
1/4 tsp.	Cayenne pepper
3 tbsp.	White miso
1	Avocado (Haas or Bacon)
1 1/2 cups	Purified water

For Garnish:

2 tbsp.	Toasted nori (crushed on top of the soup)
1/2	Vine ripened tomato, chopped
1/2 cup	Cilantro, diced
1/2 cup	Green onions, chopped

Directions:

Blend all ingredients together in your blender, until you have reached the consistency you like. We like it a little thicker than thinner. Garnish with chopped tomatoes, cilantro and green onions and toasted Nori. Just place Nori sheets over the top of your gas or electric burner and toast until it starts to shrink up. Be very careful.

Linda's Tips:

Love this recipe and would highly recommend using this soup for a three day purifying cleanse, along with any of our Digestive Juice Aids located on pages 20-21

Prep Time: 10m | Serving: 2 | 100% Living

29. Our Living Fruit Soup

Ingredients:

1 cup	Our Living Granola (recipe #51)
2 cups	Frozen berries such as: strawberries, blueberries, blackberries or Acai fruit
1/4 cup	Pure water

Directions:

Blend the following ingredients in a high powered blender:
Berries and water. (if it's too watery, add one banana)
Put berries puree, (which is what it should look like) into a bowl
Top with Our Living Granola.
End with topping sliced bananas and other fruit sliced such as pears and or apples to finish it off.

Linda's Tips:

This makes for a great summer soup and it is so good. I put this recipe into our Living Soup section, but it's really good for breakfast and can be used as an after-noon soup, as well. The berries are very low on the glycemic scale, so anyone with sugar issues such as hypoglycemia can tolerate this recipe. Plus berries are incredibly healthy for good brain function. Berries are available year round in frozen form, so you can use this recipe any time of year Try to find Acai frozen fruit-it's worth it.

.

Kids love this recipe too.

Pate's - Dips - Spreads and Toppings

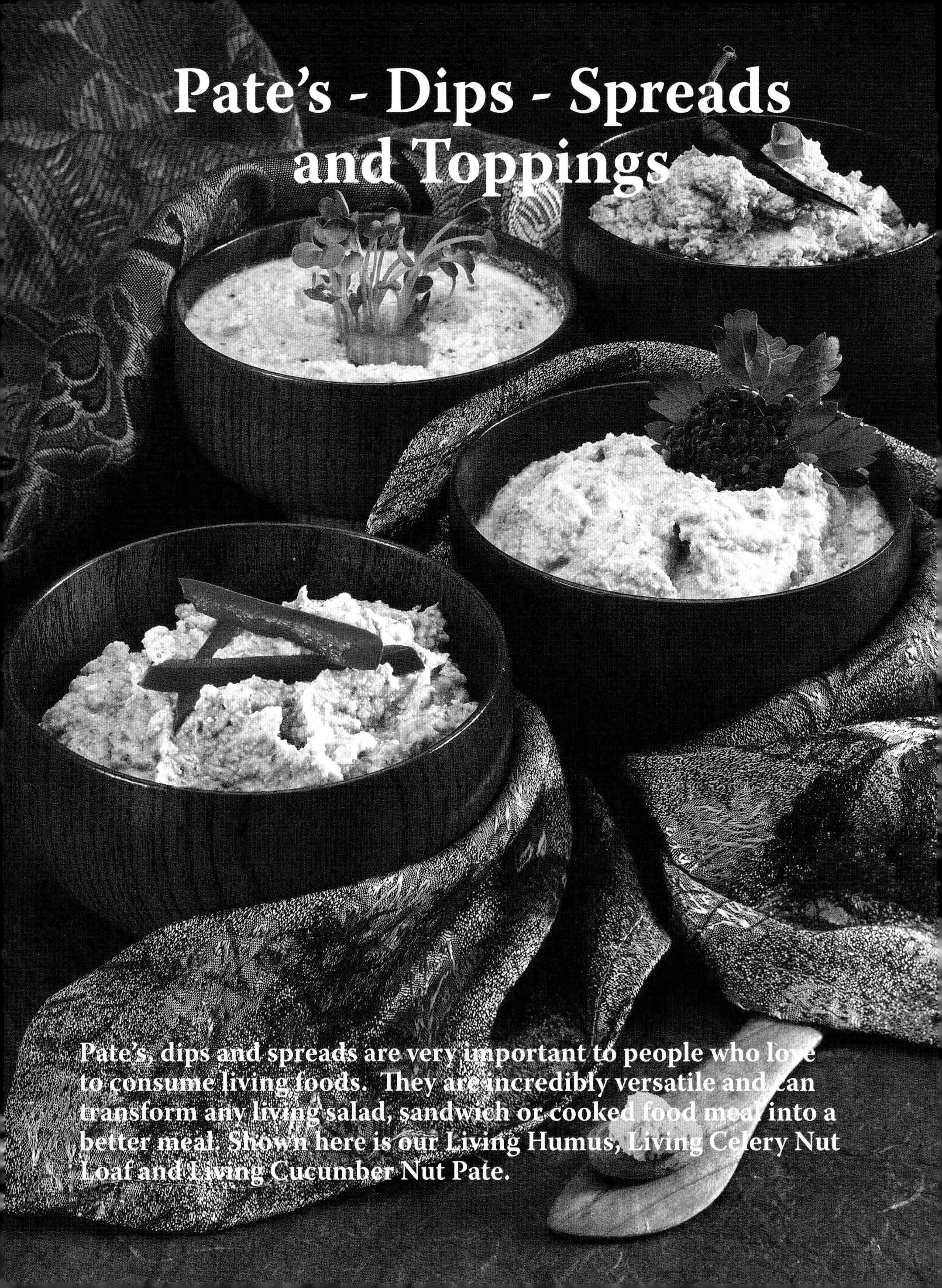

Pate's, dips and spreads are very important to people who love to consume living foods. They are incredibly versatile and can transform any living salad, sandwich or cooked food meal into a better meal. Shown here is our Living Humus, Living Celery Nut Loaf and Living Cucumber Nut Pate.

Prep Time:10m · Serving: 4 · 100% Living

30. Living Humus

Ingredients:

2 cups	Sprouted garbonzo beans
3 tbsp. each	Fresh Lemon juice and lime juice
2 cloves	Garlic
1 tbsp.	Sesame tahini
1 tsp.	Cumin
2 tbsp.	Olive oil
1 tsp.	Curry powder
1/3 cup	Cilantro or parsley, diced
_ cup	Black olives
1 tsp.	Kelp
1 tsp.	Nutritional yeast
1	Pinch cumin
1/2 tsp.	Red pepper
1 tbsp.	Nama Shoyu

Salt and pepper to taste

Directions:

Put all ingredients into blender, and blend for approximately one minute.

Linda's Tip:

This is a fantastic classic dish, however with the sprouted garbonzo beans, this classic dish becomes completely alive, filled with living enzymes to help in better digestion. We usually put this on top of our salads which contain olives and onions in the salad. We also use this spread inside cabbage leaves and eat along with a full green salad such as #15 on page 128

Prep Time:5m | Serving: 2-4 | 100% Living

#31 Super Simple Guacamole

Ingredients:

4	Ripe Avocados (Haas)
3 tbsp.	Fresh lime juice
2-3 tbsp.	Diced yellow onion
one handful	Cilantro, diced (optional)

Sea salt and pepper to taste

Directions:

Mash avocados, then add lime juice, onion and use sea salt and pepper to taste.

Linda's Tips:

This easy to prepare dip works well as a topping over our World Tostada located on page 214, recipe #92.

✿Prep Time:10m ✿ Serving: 4 ✿ 80% Living

#32 Eggless Tofu Mayonnaise

Ingredients:

1 pkg.	Extra firm organic silken tofu
1 1/2 tbsp.	Cider vinegar or fresh lemon juice
1 tsp.	Succanant, stevia or honey
1 tsp.	Sea salt
1/2 tsp.	Dry mustard
1/8 tsp.	White pepper

Directions:

In Blender, put all ingredients and blend until smooth.

Linda's Tips:

This recipe can last up to a few weeks. Great used as a spread or as an addition to a dressing to make it creamier.

Prep Time:10m | Serving: 4 | 100% Living

33. Our Favorite Simple Salsa

Ingredients

3 cups	Vine ripened tomatoes or Roma tomatoes, diced
1/2 cup	Fresh cilantro, diced
1/2 cup	Fresh parsley, minced
1/4 cup	Yellow onion, diced
1	Large clove, garlic, crushed
2	Limes or lemons, juiced either through juicer, or by hand
2 tsp.	Jalapeno pepper, minced
1/2 tsp.	Sea salt to taste

Directions:

Chop and dice all ingredients and place into a dish for immediate consumption! This recipe goes great with our World Tostada (put over the top) and on top of our living soups, and on top of our basic cooked salads.

Linda's Tips:

We love this recipe with our simple guacamole recipe #31 listed on page 146, and #90 on page 212, our Tofu Tacos. Sometimes in the summertime we mix our regular red tomatoes we use in this recipe with those beautiful heirloom tomatoes that are either orange, yellow or red. Enjoy!

Prep Time:15m | Serving: 3 | 100% Living

34. Living Celery Nut Loaf

Ingredients:

5	Stalks celery
1 cup	Almonds, soaked overnight
1	Haas avocado
3 tbsps.	Onion, chopped
3 tbsps.	Parsley
1	Medium lemon, juiced
l/2 tsp.	Sage
l/4 tsp.	Paprika
1 tbsp.	Jensen's seasoning,Tamari or brown miso.

Directions:

Homogenize in order (blender, food processor or champion) almonds, avocado, and one stalk celery. Repeat. Shape into loaf with your hands, or use as a pate, or use on top of your salad, or use in sandwiches as a spread.

Linda's Tips:

Make sure the almonds are soaked overnight, otherwise, it's very hard to blend and it makes the loaf very dry. Lasts about two days in the refrigerator.

✽Prep Time10m: ✽ Serving: 3 ✽ 100% Living

35. Living Cucumber Nut Pate

Ingredients:

1	Cucumber, peeled
1 cup	Sunflower Seeds
1	Large clove garlic, crushed
l/4	yellow or sweet onion
2 tsps.	Cajun seasoning or seasalt and black pepper to taste

Directions:

1.) Blend cucumber to a liquid consistency

2.) Soak sunflower seeds in blended cucumber overnight

3.) In the morning blend the sunflower/cucumber mix with the remaining ingredients (garlic, onion and spices)

Linda's Tips:

Serve as a sandwich spread or use on top of really any salad, or as a spread over our flax seed cracker recipe # 54 located on page 172

Prep Time:10m ✿ Serving: 4-6 ✿ 60-75% Living

36. Homemade Humus

Ingredients:

1 cup	Cooked garbanzo beans
l/2 lb.	Firm organic tofu
3	Large cloves garlic
1/4 cup	Fresh lemon juice
2 tsp.	Sesame tahini
l/4 cup	Fresh parsley or cilantro
1 tbsp.	Paprika or chili powder
2 tsp.	Sea salt
1 tsp.	Black pepper

Directions:

1. Blend all ingredients together except paprika in blender or food processor until creamy.
2. Sprinkle paprika over top as a garnish

Linda's Tips:

Will last in the refrigerator for 7 days, but we only keep it for 5. Great as a spread in a sandwich, topping on a salad, use as a pate or dip, or eat as a snack with our flax cracker recipe # 54 on page 172, and/or recipe #53 on page 171. Sprinkle a little paprika, parsley and cilantro, diced finely for a nice green addition for the top of the humus. Drizzle a little organic olive oil on top. These additions make your humus really come alive! Also good on top of our Basic Salad recipe #1a on page 113.

Our Super Salad Dressings and Sauces

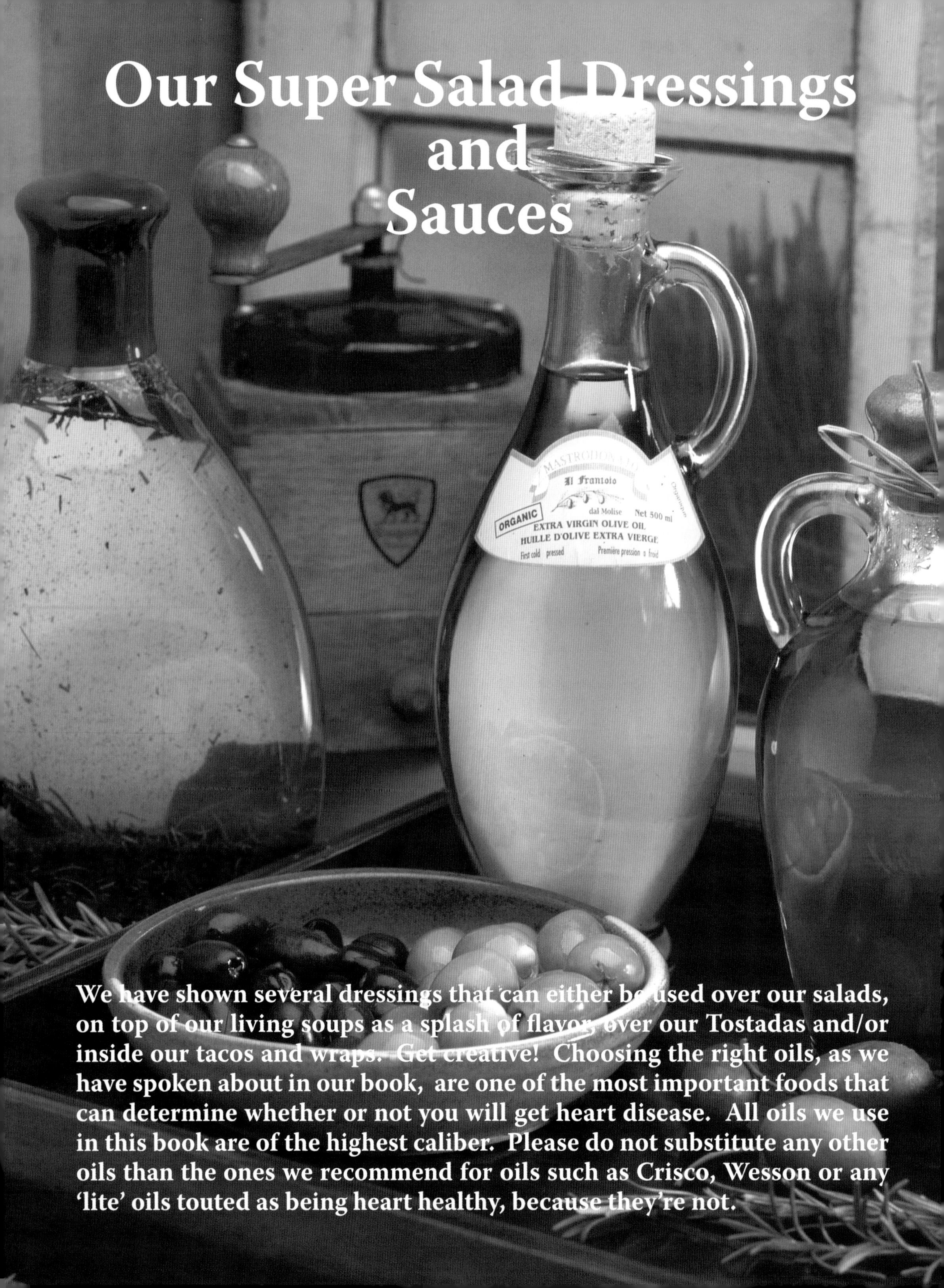

We have shown several dressings that can either be used over our salads, on top of our living soups as a splash of flavor, over our Tostadas and/or inside our tacos and wraps. Get creative! Choosing the right oils, as we have spoken about in our book, are one of the most important foods that can determine whether or not you will get heart disease. All oils we use in this book are of the highest caliber. Please do not substitute any other oils than the ones we recommend for oils such as Crisco, Wesson or any 'lite' oils touted as being heart healthy, because they're not.

✽Prep Time: 5m ✽Serving: 4 ✽ 100% Living

37. Tofu Tarragon Tomato

Ingredients:

1	Medium-large vine ripened tomato
1/4 cup	Apple Cider vinegar
1 tsp.	Freshly ground black pepper
2 tbsps.	Fresh Tarragon
1/2 tsp.	Organic seasalt
1/2 cup	Organic olive oil
2 cloves	Organic garlic
1 tsp.	Organic mustard
3 tbsps.	Organic tofu (soft or medium)
Pinch	Red Pepper or Cayenne

Directions:

Blend all ingredients, except the oil, in a blender. While continuing to blend ingredients, slowly drizzle in oil until dressing thickens.

Linda's Tips:

Good over recipe #13 on page 136, our Mid-Eastern Salad.

Prep Time:5m | Serving: 4 | 100% Living

38. Heartsmart Omega 3 Dressing

Ingredients:

1/3 cup	Flax oil
1/2 cup	Olive oil
1/4 cup	Rice vinegar or apple cider vinegar
1 tbsp.	Honey
1 tbsp.	Fresh minced basil
1 tbsp.	Fresh minced tarragon
1 tbsp.	Minced fresh oregano
4	Clove garlic
1 1/2 tsp.	Spike season or cajun seasoning

Dash of black pepper

Directions:

Blend in blender until liquefied.

Linda's Tips:

You can substitute other fresh herbs of your choice to change tastes. We suggest adding fresh parsley, cilantro in place of tarragon and basil for a change.

Prep Time: 5m | Serving: 4 | 100% Living

39. Royal Thai Salad Dressing

Ingredients:

1 cup	Orange juice, freshly squeezed
1/4 cup	Rice vinegar
1 tsp.	Ginger
1 tsp.	Garlic
1 tbsp.	Nama shoyu
2 tbsp.	Toasted sesame oil
Pinch	Cayenne pepper

Directions:

Blend all ingredients together. Refrigerate for up to five days.

Linda's Tips:

Great with Asian oriented salads such as #18 on page 131.

Prep Time:5m | Serving: 4 | 100% Living

40. Fresh Herb Salad Dressing

Ingredients:

1 cup	Olive Oil or unrefined Grape seed Oil
2 cloves	Garlic
1/3 cup	Yellow onion
1/2 cup	Fresh spinach
1/2 cup	Fresh parsley
1/2 cup	Fresh cilantro
3/4 cup	Fresh dill
1 tbsp.	Tamari
2 tbsp.	Balsamic Vinegar or Apple Cider Vinegar
1/2 cup	Pure water (more or less depending on the consistency you like.)

Dash cayenne pepper

Directions:

Blend water and all ingredients except oil in a blender.
Slowly add in the oil to help emulsify the oil into the dressing.

Linda's Tip:

This is a wonderful light green dressing to go over vegetarian tacos on page 210, recipe #88 or poured over any of our living soups to give it a nice oily consistency.

Prep Time:5-10m | Serving: 2 | 80% Living

41. Superfast Tofu Dressing

Ingredients:

1/2 lb.	Organic tofu, soft
2 tbsps.	Fresh lemon juice
2 tbsps.	Organic olive oil
1/2 tsp.	Sea salt
1/8 tsp.	Ground black pepper
1 tbsp.	Fresh parsley or Cilantro
1	Clove garlic

Directions:

1) Blend and serve!

Linda's Tip:

Great dressing over salads, especially salads with nuts or seeds in them such as salad # 12, page 125. Our kids love them as a veggie dip or over steamed veggies and rice.

Prep Time: 5m | Serving: 4 | 100% Living

42. Super Green Salad Dressing

Ingredients:

2 cloves	Garlic, freshly pressed
1/2 cup	Fresh organic olive oil
1/4 cup	Chopped scallions (green onions)
2 tbsp.	Fresh lemon juice
4 tbsp.	Apple cider vinegar
1/4 cup	Parsley
1/4 cup	Cilantro
1/4 cup	Spinach
1 tsp.	Fresh organic tarragon
1 tsp.	Sea salt

Black pepper and red pepper to taste

Directions:

1). Add all ingredients together, except the oil.
2). Blend the oil in slowly to make sure the dressing emulsifies correctly.

Linda's Tips:

This is a great salad dressing-full of antioxidants with the abundance of greens. This is a great dressing for the summertime

Prep Time: 5m | Serving: 4 | 100% Living

43. Macadamia Oil Dressing

Ingredients:

1/2 cup	Olive or macadamia oil
1 tsp.	Organic dijon mustard
2 tbsp.	Fresh lemon juice
4 tbsp.	Apple cider vinegar
1/4 cup	Parsley
1/4 cup	Cilantro
1/4 cup	Spinach
1 tsp.	Sea salt

Black pepper and red pepper to taste

Directions:

1). Add all ingredients together, except the oil.
2). Blend the oil in slowly to make sure the dressing emulsifies correctly.

Linda's Tips:

This is a great salad dressing-full of antioxidants with the abundance of greens. This is a great dressing for the summertime and drizzled on top of any of our living soups, and over the top of our Tofu Tacos, recipe # 90 on page 212.

Prep Time: 5m | **Serving: 2** | **100% Living**

44. Superfast Tahini Dressing

Ingredients:

2 tbsps.	Miso (brown)
1/4 cup	Organic Tahini
1 small	Clove Garlic
1/4 cup	Fresh lemon juice
1 Pinch	Cayenne Pepper

Directions:

Blend all together slowly and serve! You may want to add water to achieve the consistency you like. Thicker makes for a good sauce over steamed vegetables, and thinner makes for a better salad dressing.

Linda's Tips:

This is the greatest dressing when you are tired and need a fresh dressing right away. It's a real winner and the entire family loves this recipe. This versatile recipe also goes GREAT over living soups.

Prep Time:5m | Serving: 4 | 100% Living

45. No Fat Herb Dressing

Ingredients:

3/4 cup	Fresh tomato juice
1/4 cup	Apple cider vinegar
1 tbsp.	Fresh parsley
1 tbsp.	Chopped chives or green scallions
1	Clove fresh garlic
l/2 tsp.	Sea salt
1	Pinch dried oregano
1/4 tsp	Honey or stevia for sweetness
1	Pinch cayenne
1	Pinch freshly ground black pepper to taste

Directions:

1). Blend in blender all ingredients until liquefied. Will last for 5 days in refrigerator.

Linda's Tips:

Remember stevia comes in a liquid form, so we need to make sure when you use the stevia, it's only about l/2 tsp. However the sucanant is in powdered form, so you may just want to use about a tsp.

This is a great dressing when you want to cut the fat out of our diet for a few weeks to lose weight, or you may use this dressing over your salad, and use another source of fat inside the salad such as avocados. This way, only a small portion of your salad contains fat.

Prep Time: 5m | Serving: 4 | 75% Living

46.Sundried Tomato Tahini Dressing

Ingredients:

2 tbsp.	Sesami tahini
1 1/2 tsp.	White or brown miso
2 tsp.	Lemon or lime juice
1 clove	Garlic
1/2 tsp.	Red pepper flakes
1/2 cup	Water
6 tbsp.	Extra virgin olive oil
8	Sun-dried tomatoes
1 tsp.	Sea salt or 1 tsp. nama shoyu

Directions:

Store the sun-dried tomatoes overnight in the 6 tbsp. of olive oil. Place entire ingredients into the blender except for the water and blend for at least one to two minutes to make sure all the ingredients are liquefied. Slowly add the water into the dressing.

Linda's Tips:

You may make this dressing as thick or thin as you like by adding more or less water. Since we enjoy using this also as a spread over steamed vegetables or inside a veggie-burger, or our Nutty Rice and Veggies recipe # 83, page 205 or recipe #86, located on page 208, our Perfect Pita Sandwich. Sometimes we make it a bit thicker by not putting as much water as recommended. Otherwise, as a dressing, it's great just as it is displayed in the recipe.

✿Prep Time: 5m ✿Serving: 4 ✿ 100% Living

47. Carrot Juice Veggie Dressing

Ingredients:

1/2 cup	Freshly made carrot juice
2 tsp.	Fresh unpasteurized miso
2 tbsp.	Organic sesame tahini
1	Medium sized clove garlic
1	Tomato, medium sized
1/2	Red bell pepper
1/2 tsp.	Jalapeno pepper
1/2 tsp.	Fresh tarragon
1/3 cup	Organic olive oil
2 tbsp.	Fresh lemon or lime juice

Handful of parsley and cilantro, juiced

Sea salt and pepper to taste

Directions:

Alternate juicing the carrots and greens together, so to make sure the carrots flush out the greens as you are juicing, because carrots have a lot more juice in them than greens, and sometimes the greens get stuck inside the bowl of the juicer. This is why alternating the carrots with the greens is such a good idea. Combine all ingredients except for the olive oil, and blend until liquefied (approximately one minute). Slowly add in the olive oil.

Linda's Tips:

This is a phyto-chemically rich salad dressing, and used best in salads that contain nuts, seeds and/or a salad rich in diversity with shredded vegetables, for example: recipe #8, on page 120.

Our Living Breakfasts

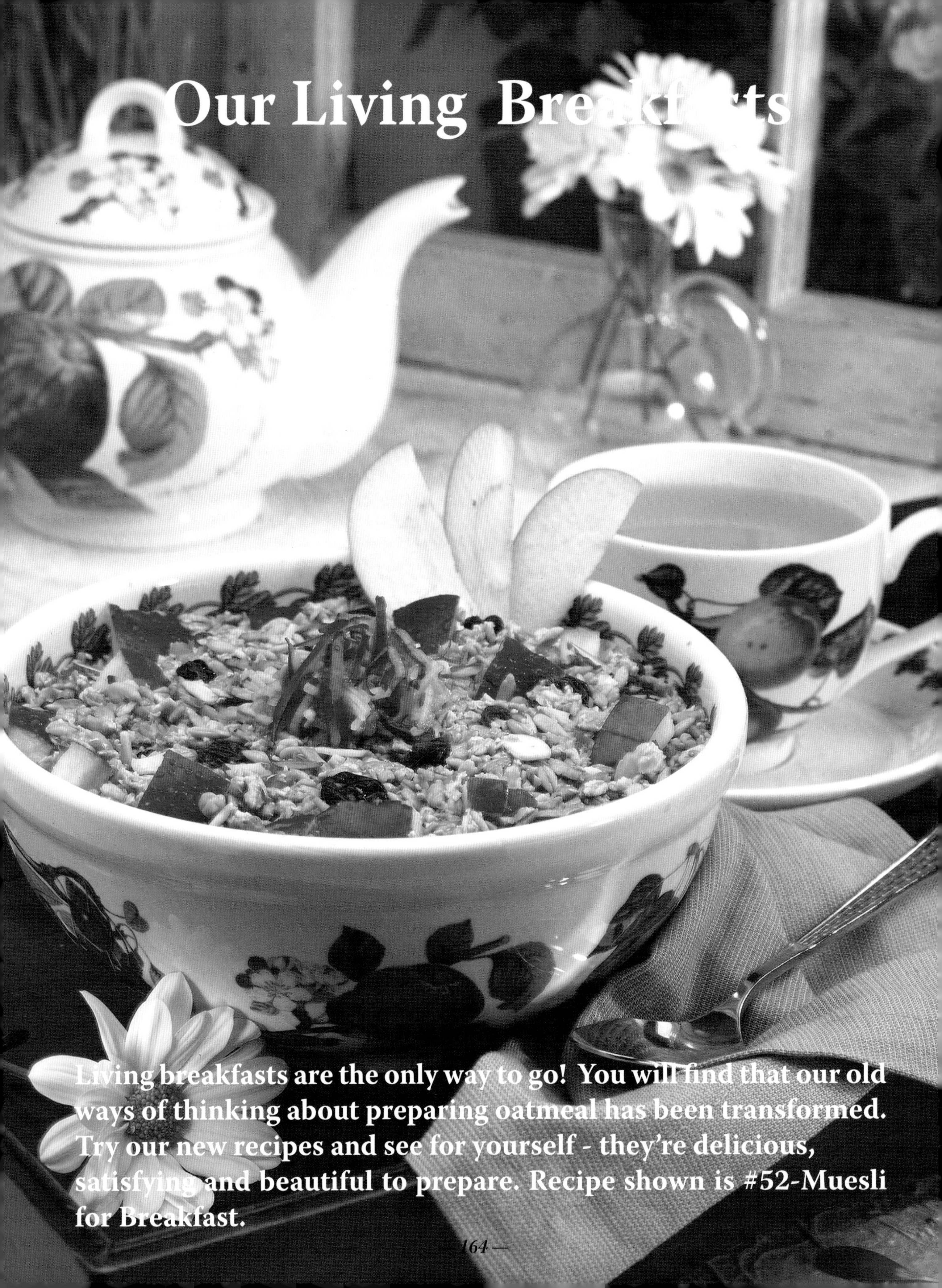

Living breakfasts are the only way to go! You will find that our old ways of thinking about preparing oatmeal has been transformed. Try our new recipes and see for yourself - they're delicious, satisfying and beautiful to prepare. Recipe shown is #52-Muesli for Breakfast.

Prep Time: 20m   Serving: 6   100% Living

48. Breakfast Pie

Ingredients:

1 lb.	Organic strawberries
1/2 cup	Organic Macadamia nuts
1 tsp.	Nutmeg
1/2 tsp.	Cinnamon
1 tbsp.	Organic Honey
1	Young Baby Coconut (and its water)
1/2 cup	Organic dates
1 1/2 cup	Sunflower Seeds
2	Bananas, peeled
3	Kiwis, peeled

Directions:

1.) Blend in blender the following: strawberries, coconut, liquid and-macadamia nuts, honey, nutmeg and cinnamon until thick enough for a dressing over your beautiful new pie. (Refrigerate one hour)

2.) In a food processor: Blend dates and sunflower seeds for approximately two minutes in the food processor. Within time your crust will start to get a bit warm as you witness it continuing to process. As soon as you see the crust start to clump up a bit, stop.

3.) Now your crust is ready to form onto the pie shell. 11 inch pie shell is fine. We recommend glass only.

4.) Form crust from the dates and sunflower seeds. Let stand in the refrigerator for about 10 minutes while you are arranging your strawberries, kiwis and bananas to be prepared and sliced for the pie.

5.) When you are ready to form the pie with the fruit, take the glass pie shell out of the refrigerator and begin to layer the bottom of the pie shell with bananas, then kiwis and then strawberries. Continue this way leaving the strawberries on the top when finished.

6.) Top with the strawberry cream and refrigerate for one hour. Now your living pie is ready!

7.) Make this recipe the night before, so your fruit pie is ready for breakfast, and this kind of pie will last 24-48 hours.

Prep Time:10m | Serving: 4 | 100% Living

49. Apricot and Almond Delight

Ingredients:

1/2 cup	Slivered almonds
2/3 cup	Dried, organic apricots (soak 1 hour before)
2 cups	Whole rolled oats (soaked 30 minutes before)
1 cup	Flax seeds
1/2 cup	Hemp seeds
1/2 cup	Organic raisins
1/3 cup	Organic pumpkin seeds (raw and crushed)
1 cup	Fruit of the season, sliced, to be placed on top

Honey, vanilla, nutmeg or cinnamon drizzled on top.

Use fresh almond milk, macadamia nut milk or banana milk as a substitute for regular milk.

Directions:

Add all ingredients together and enjoy! Makes for a great breakfast cereal full of proteins, fats and complex carbohydrates.

Linda's Tips:

For a great protein rush in the morning, this is a great recipe. I particularly like this recipe in the winter by using freshly chopped pears and apples as a topping, and if I'm in a sour mood, crush some fresh cranberries in for good measure.

We use fresh almond milk usually, but you can substitute store bought organic soy milk if you're in a pinch. Remember to top with honey.

✿Prep Time:15m ✿Serving:12 ✿ 100% Living

50. Loving Living Granola

Ingredients:

2 cups	Steel cut oats
1/2 cup	Macadamia nuts, chopped
1/2 cup	Sunflower seeds
1 cup	Regular oats
1/2 cup	Walnuts, chopped
1/3 cup	Organic sesame seeds
1/3 cup	Organic hemp seeds
1/2 cup	Almonds, slivered or crushed
1/2 cup	Shredded coconuts
1/2 cup	Organic raisins
1/2 cup	Dried cranberries

Directions:

Place the oats onto a dehydrator sheet and drizzle honey over the top. Dehydrate for approximately 8 hours at 105 degrees, or on very low heat in the oven for only 1 hour. Place all the oats into a bowl with the rest of the ingredients. Mix well and keep in dry place for up to two months. (Raisins and cranberries are natural preservatives).

Linda's Tips:

We love, love love this recipe! Fantastic for wintertime and springtime for breakfast. Great protein breakfast and an overall fantastic breakfast. Don't forget to add a lot of fresh seasonal fruit on top. Use our fresh nut milks located on page 75, 76 and 77 for a dreamy breakfast.

Prep Time: 15m | Serving: 10 | 100% Living

51. It's Alive! Living Granola

Ingredients:

5 cups	Organic regular oats
1 cup	Walnuts (raw)
1 cup	Almonds (raw)
1/2 cup	Sunflower Seeds (raw)
1/2 cup	Pumpkin Seeds (raw)
1 cup	Organic, plump raisins
1/2 cup	Grated coconut flakes
1/2 cup	Organic Flax and sesame seeds
1/2 tsp. each	Cinnamon, anise, nutmeg

Toppings: Fresh Berries and Bananas in spring/summertime stone fruits-without stone (fall and wintertime use shredded apples and pears and blueberries)

Directions:

Put the oats into a very large bowl so the rest of the ingredients can be added to it: Add: chopped walnuts and almonds. Then add the sunflower seeds, pumpkin seeds, flax seeds and sesame seeds, raisins, and coconut flakes. Follow through with the cinnamon, anise and nutmeg spices . This recipe will last in the refrigerator for at least two weeks, without of course, any liquids put into them.

Linda's Tips:

For breakfast or snack: Put granola into bowl, and then add our favorite recipe # 56 57, or 58 on page 175-177 for fresh nutmilks, or use organic soy milk. Let sit for approximately ten to fifteen minutes before eating so as to soften the oats.

✽Prep Time: 5m ✽ Serving: 2 ✽ 100% Living

52. Muesli for Breakfast

Ingredients:

1 cup	Steel cut oats
1 cup	Pure water
1/2 cup	Raisins
1/2 cup	Pitted prunes or dates, chopped
1/2 cup	Dried apricots, chopped
1/2 cup	Apple, grated
1/4 cup	Raw organic almonds, slivered
3 tbsp.	Organic honey

Directions:

In a large mixing bowl, combine all the ingredients and mix well. Cover and place in refrigerator overnight. Remove muesli for 1 hour before serving. This cereal makes for outstanding nutritional breakfast.

Linda's Tips:

We highly recommend eating three different types of fruits over the top of this breakfast that's in season. Samples would be: fall/wintertime: blueberries, apples, pears and fuyu persimmons. Spring/Summertime would be: strawberries, other berries, stone fruits such as nectarines, peaches and other fruits such as, good old year round bananas!

Our Living Breads

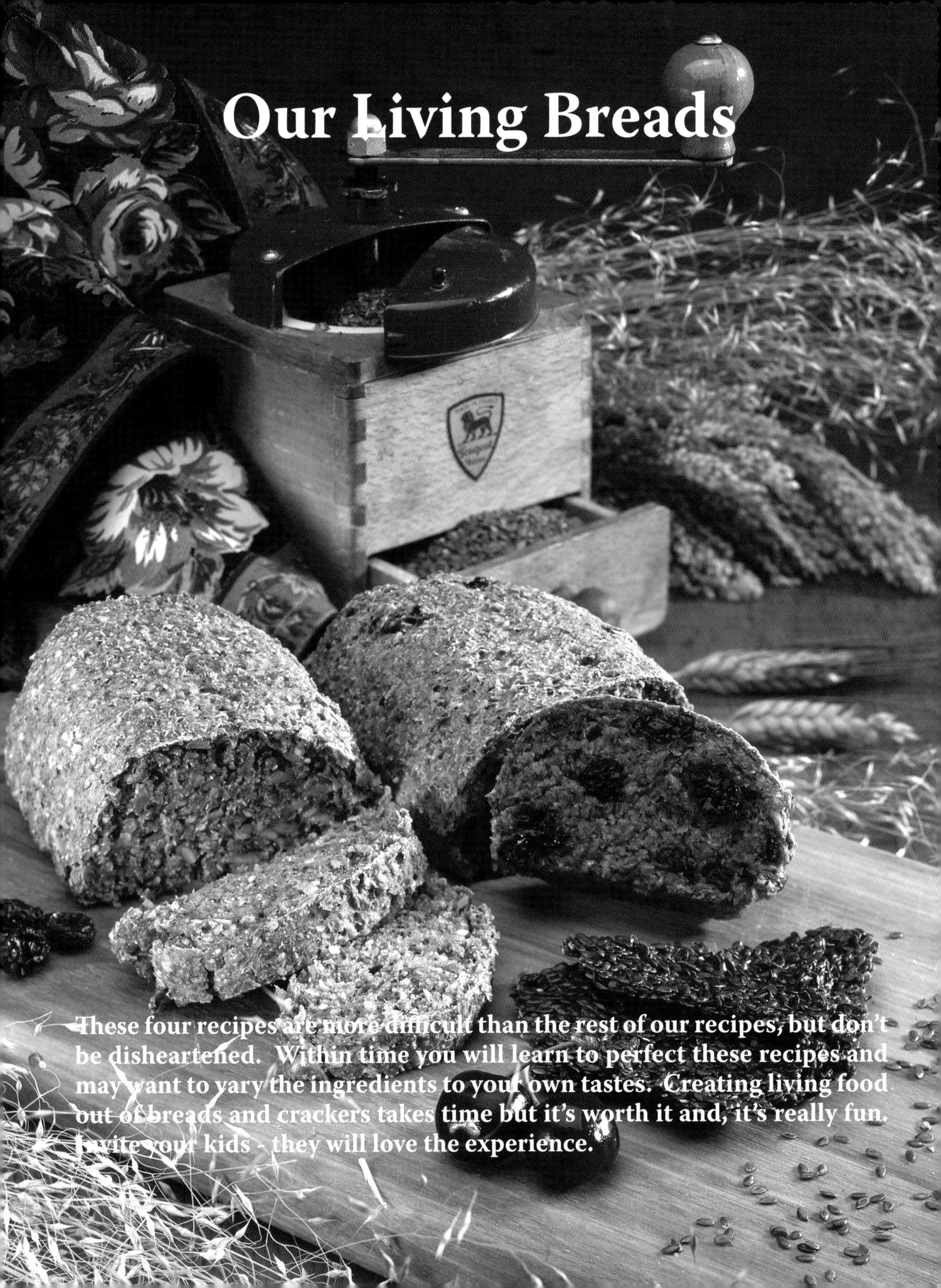

These four recipes are more difficult than the rest of our recipes, but don't be disheartened. Within time you will learn to perfect these recipes and may want to vary the ingredients to your own tastes. Creating living food out of breads and crackers takes time but it's worth it and, it's really fun. Invite your kids - they will love the experience.

✽ Prep Time:1hour ✽ Serving: 4 ✽ 100% Living

53. Living Essene Bread

Ingredients:

2 cups	Sprouted wheat berries*
1/2 cup	Chopped dates
1/4 cup	Sunflower seeds (raw)
1/2 cup	Soaked raisins (8 hours)

Directions:

1. Sprout your wheat berries overnight (place in a glass jar filled with purified water.) Rinse three times per day with fresh water, in a dark room for 24 hours, or until their sprouts are about 1/4 inch long. Rinse three times per day with fresh water.

2. Stir all ingredients together. Use a champion juicer with the blank screen or use a vita mix blender to blend all ingredients.

3. Form into loaves (not more than 1 1/2 inches thick and dehydrate 12-16 hours. You can form into 2 small loaves.

Bread should be crunchy on the outside and chewy on the inside.

Linda's Tips:

This is a difficult recipe, but Jay and I wanted you to experiment and get the hang of it, rather than to keep purchasing breads that are filled with mono-dygliceries, yeasts and dough conditions that are bloating and toxic. Best to try and within time you will become an expert! These are the only breads we consistently use in our home, besides pita breads (which are yeast less), but they are still cooked at high temperatures, unlike our Living Essence Bread. This recipe goes fantastic with all of our living soups located on pages 137-143. All of our smoothies added to our Living Essene Bread is a great combination. Our smoothies are located on pages 179-185.

Prep Time: 30m   Serving: 4   100% Living

54. Basic Flax Crackers

Ingredients:

2 cups	Flax Seeds (dark brown or golden brown)
2 cups	Purified water
2 tbsp.	Soy sauce or tamari

Salt and Cayenne pepper to taste

Directions:

Soak flax seeds in the 2 cups purified water (about 8 cups purified water) overnight. (apprx. 8-12 hours). (They will expand almost double in size) Make sure to soak the seeds in a darker area where there is not a lot of light. Soak the seeds in a container that has a plate under it, as it may foam over the top. all those enzymes are at work! After soaking is accomplished, mix in the tamari, cayenne and sea salt. Spread on dehydrator sheets that come with the dehydrator. We have the Excaliber dehydrator (the texflex sheets came with the machine.) Sheets are important because the flax seeds must be able to dry and stick to the sheets so they can dry properly and be able to separate easily.
Cook at 115 degrees overnight or approximately 8 hours on each side, or until they are completely dry, so you can cut them into pieces either with your hands or carefully with a large knife that is at least six inches in length.

Linda's Tips:

These crackers are FANTASTIC for living soups, dips, and cracked over salads.
Flax crackers are one of the most powerful changes we can make
to our diets that will show quick results in energy and bowel improvements. Also, you can add all kinds of different herbs and spices to this basic recipe, including tomatoes for a really nice variety of crackers.

Prep Time:1hour | Serving: 4 | 100% living

55. Tomato-Herb Flax Crackers

Ingredients:

2 cups	Flax seeds
1/2	Onion
4 large	Cloves garlic
1 cup	Sundried tomatoes
2 tsp.	Italian seasoning
2 large	Basil leaves
4 tbsp.	Tamari or nama shoyu
Pinch of Seasalt	

Directions:

Soak flax seeds overnight (they will double in size overnight)

Soak tomatoes and onions overnight in purified water or for 4 hours.

Then blend in blender (save the water-you may need it) blend onions and tomatoes, herbs and all seasonings. Use the saved water if you need it for blending. In a large bowl, add the mixture to the flax seeds that have been soaking from overnight. Use your spatula to spread evenly over the texflex sheets on your dehydrator.

Then take a knife and score the flax cracker mixture that is now on your texflex sheets into squares - approximately 24. If you want bigger crackers, then we suggest cutting them into 12, or vice versa.

Dehydrate at 110 for about 6 hours, then flip over to bake another 6-8. Leave sit overnight. Within 24 hours, they should be completely read to eat.

This recipe makes about 45-50- crackers and last several weeks if you keep them fresh in a container.

Linda's Tips:

This is a great recipe and makes for great bowel results if you have trouble with constipation. Now that we have that out of the way, did I tell you they taste great? Well, they do and you will love to eat them with our living soup recipes located on pages 137-143. They are also wonderful crushed into our Basic Salad #1 on page 113, (or any other whole meal salad). If you want more fiber for your living granola recipe # 50 and 51, try sprinkling them over the top.

Our Living Nut Milks

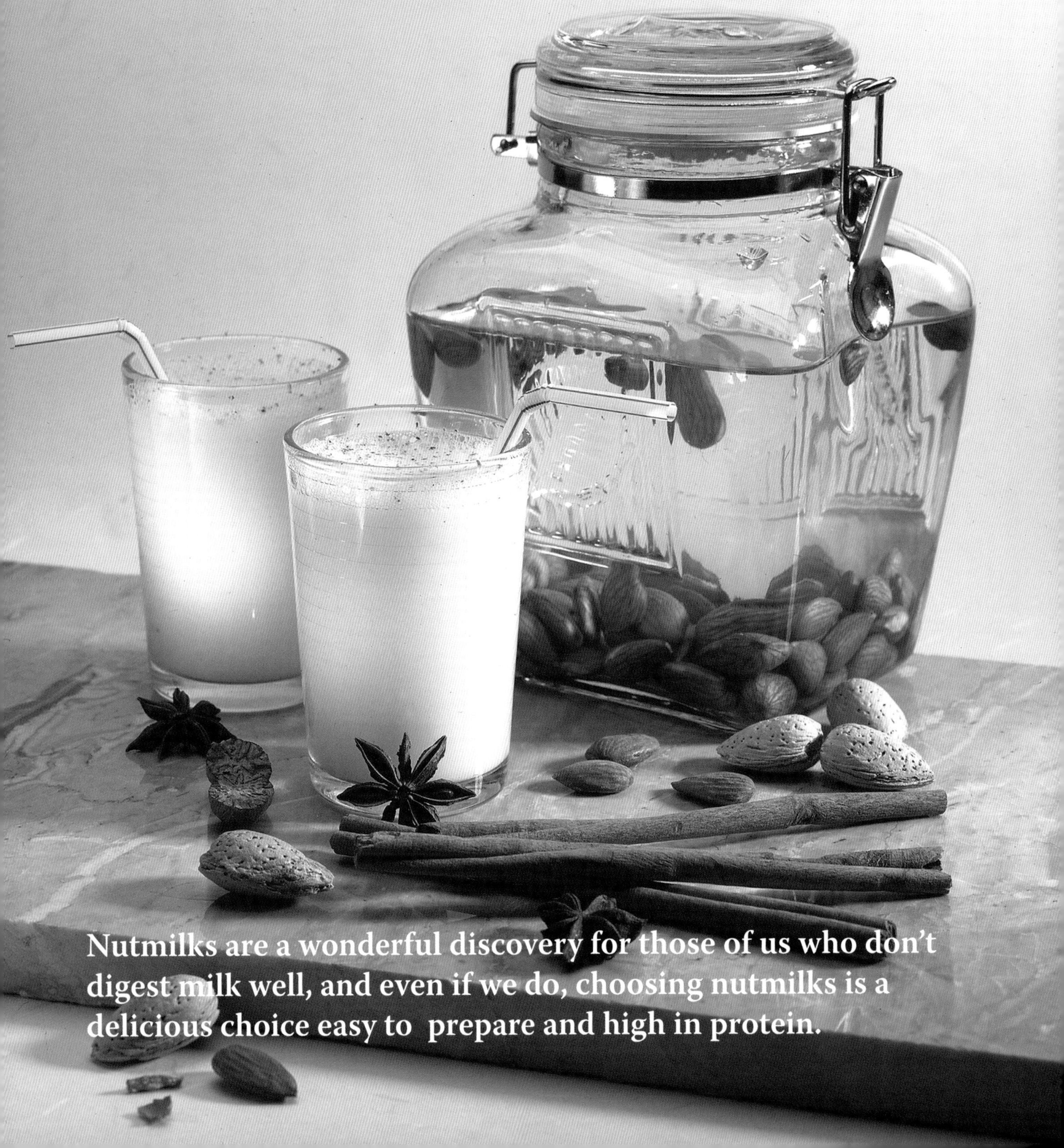

Nutmilks are a wonderful discovery for those of us who don't digest milk well, and even if we do, choosing nutmilks is a delicious choice easy to prepare and high in protein.

✿ Prep Time: 5m ✿Serving: 4 ✿ 100% Living

56. Living Almond Milk

Ingredients

1 cups	Organic Almonds (raw)
4 cups	Purified Water
1 tbsp.	Organic Vanilla extract
3	Dates (pitted)

Directions:

Soak almonds overnight. In the morning, place soaked almonds and water into a hi-speed or professional blender. For thinner, less pulpy almond milk, see Jay's Tips below.

With any of your seed milks, add frozen berries and ice (to your tasting) We usually add about 1/2 cup strawberries, blueberries, boysenberries or cranberries and when pomegranates are in season we add those too. With the cranberries and pomegranates add more honey to the recipe to keep it from being too bitter.
This recipe makes an incredible smoothie that's out of this world!

Jay's Tips:

Almond milk will last approximately 3 days in the refrigerator. Almond milk is a wonderful substitute for any kind of dish asking for milk, although remember it is a bit nutty in flavor, and has small residues of pulp, unless you strain it with a cheesecloth before consuming. This is easily done by using a cheesecloth after liquefying all ingredients. Pour almond milk (which should still be a bit warm) into the cheese cloth, and slowly squeeze milk through. Residue can be kept for recipes for smoothies such as recipe # 59 on page 179, but this would be strictly for fiber only, as the milky part of the nut has been removed. This almond milk recipes goes wonderfully with recipes Loving Living Granola, It's Alive Living Granola and/or Muesli for Breakfast - recipe# 50, 51 or recipe #52, on pages 167, 168, 169.

Prep Time: 15m | Serving: 4 | 100% Living

57. Living Macadamia Milk

Ingredients:

1 cup	Macadamia nuts (raw)
3 cups	Purified Water
1 tsp.	Vanilla extract, organic
1 tbsp.	Honey

Directions:

Soak the macadamia nuts at overnight or at least 4 hours before blending. (Do not use the water from the macadamia nuts while it was soaking.) Once you discard the soaked water, add all ingredients into blender, and liquefy until it starts to take on a milky consistency. Not necessary to strain, but if you want the consistency to be more clear like real milk, then we recommend using a cheesecloth to push nutmilks through. Only good for one-two days in the refrigerator.

Here's a great Variation:

With any of your seed milks, add frozen berries and ice (to your tasting) We usually add about 1/2 cup strawberries, blueberries, boysenberries or cranberries and when pomegranates are in season we add those too. With the cranberries and pomegranates add more honey to the recipe to keep it from being too bitter. This recipe makes an incredible smoothie that's out of this world!

Jay's Tips:

For those who don't want to drink almond or soy milk, this is a wonderful substitute. We love this milk, when freshly made, put over recipe #49, Apricot and Almond Delight, on page 166, page 167, recipe #50, Loving Living Granola, or page 168, recipe #51, It's Alive Living Granola.

Prep Time: 15m | Serving: 4 | 100% Living

58. Living Cashew Milk

Ingredients:

1 Cup	Organic Cashews (Raw)
1 tbsp.	Honey
1 tsp.	Vanilla extract, organic
4 cups	Purified Water

Directions:

Put all ingredients into a blender. Blend until liquefied. No need to strain, unless you want it very clear. If you do, just use a cheesecloth to strain.

Here's a great Variation:

With any of your seed milks, add frozen berries and ice (to your tasting) We usually add about 1/2 cup strawberries, blueberries, boysenberries or cranberries and when pomegranates are in season we add those too. With the cranberries and pomegranates add more honey to the recipe to keep it from being too bitter. This recipe makes an incredible smoothie that's out of this world!

Jay's Tips:

For those who don't want to drink almond or soy milk, this is a wonderful substitute. We love this milk, when freshly made, put over recipe #49, Apricot and Almond Delight, on page 166, page 167, recipe #50, Loving Living Granola, or page 168, recipe #51, It's Alive Living Granola.

Our Living Smoothies

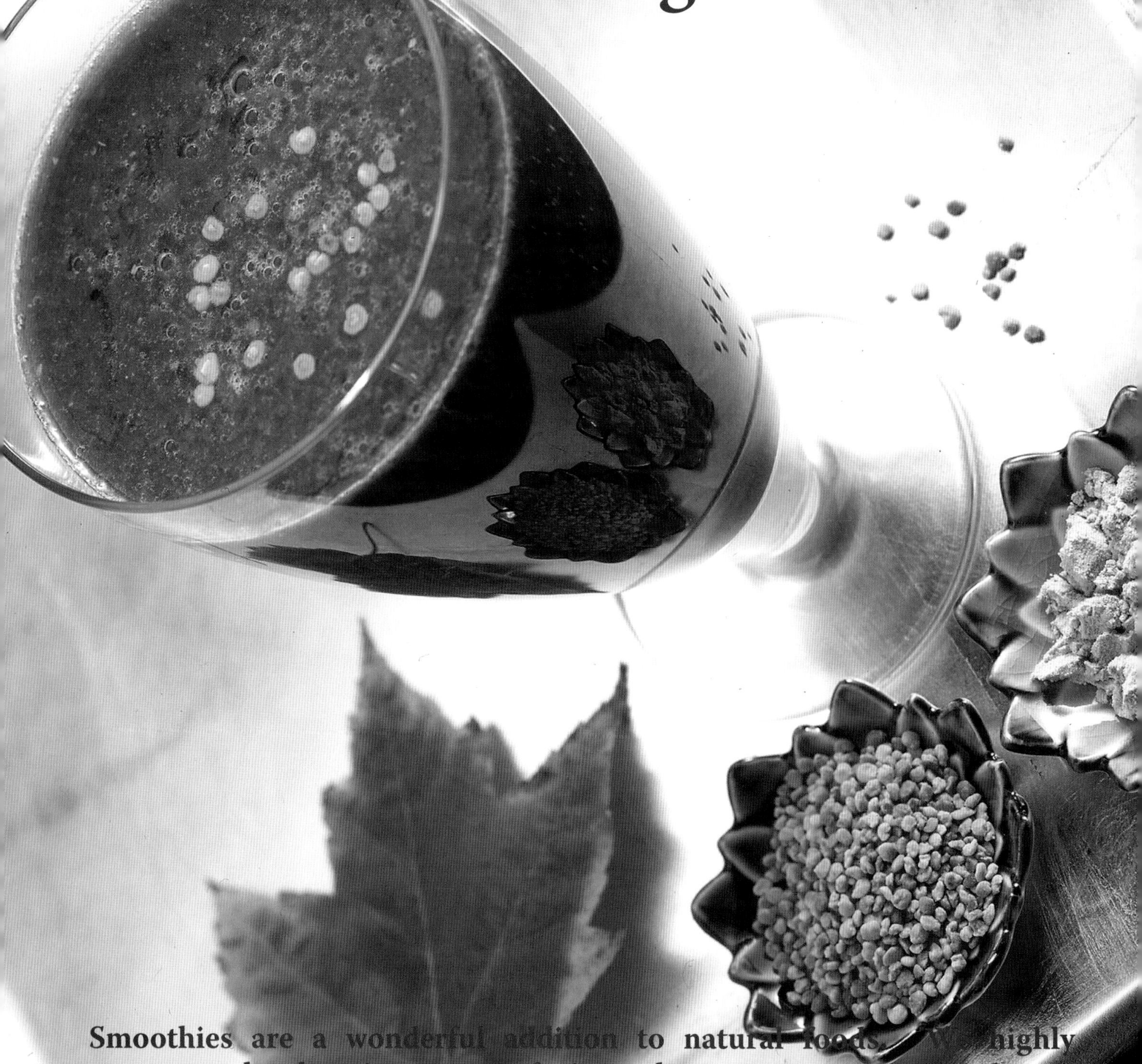

Smoothies are a wonderful addition to natural foods. We highly recommend only using organic fruits and no sweeteners, except honey on rare occasions. Children love smoothies and we recommend making them with your children. Smoothies can also be great digestive aids and great concealers for placing supergreens into. Be creative! Shown here is recipe #63- Good Morning Power up Smoothie.

Prep Time:10m | Serving: 4 | 100% Living

59. Date a Banana for Breakfast!

Ingredients:

1 cup	Fresh dates, pitted
1 1/2 cups	Freshly made almond milk (Recipe #56, page 175))
2 ripe,	Organic bananas
3/4 cup	Chopped organic walnuts

Directions:

Put dates and bananas into the blender, along with walnuts and almond milk

Another version:

Place 1/2 cup almonds and the rest of the ingredients into a professional blender, along with 1 cup ice and 1/2 cup purified water. Blend until smooth.

Linda's Tips:

Great for breakfasts whereby you will be full until later in the day, as it's very filling. For more flavor, add some liquid organic vanilla extract (1/2 tsp.)

Prep Time:5m | Serving2 | 100% Living

60. Blackberry Mama Smoothie

Ingredients:

1/2 cup	Sunflower seeds
3 1/2 cups	Pure Water
2 cups	Fresh Blackberries (frozen ok)
2	Frozen ripe Bananas
2 tbsp.	Organic Honey
1/4 tsp.	Cinnamon and nutmeg each
1 cup	Ice

Directions:

In a blender, grind sunflower seeds into a meal and slowly add water. Add the remaining ingredients and blend until smooth.

Jay's Tips:

Fantastic morning smoothie for a good protein hit in the morning. Try to use this smoothie in late summertime when Blackberries are the freshest! If not, frozen is all right too.

Prep Time: 5m | Serving2 | 100% Living

61. High Protein Nut Smoothie

Ingredients:

2 tbsp.each	Sunflower Seeds, walnuts and almonds
2 tbsp.	Flax Seeds
4 cups	Pure Water
1 cup	Fresh or frozen Berries
2 medium	Bananas, fresh or frozen
2 tbsp.	Organic Honey

Directions:

Soak the nuts for at least 15 minutes before blending. Best is to soak overnight first. Put all ingredients in hi-speed blender until liquefied.

Jay's Tips:

Great for mornings for those who run protein deficient, or hypoglycemic.

Prep Time: 10m ✽ Serving: 2 ✽ 100% Living

62. Morning Digestion Perfection

Ingredients:

1	Young baby Coconut (use the soft white coconut meat and water)
1	Orange, peeled and blended
1 inch	Fresh ginger
1/2 cup	Fresh lemon juice
Dash	Cayenne pepper to taste

Directions:

Cut open (carefully) with a cleaver, the young baby coconut, and pour the mineral water into the blender. Gently scoop out the soft coconut meat (easy to do) and place into the blender. Blend all ingredients together and drink immediately. This is a tonic, specifically designed to heal the inner lining of the stomach due to wrong eating habits, too much caffeine, alcohol or white sugared products that create digestive disturbances such as leaky gut syndrome.

Linda's Tip:

Morning is best for this drink, and try adding one tablespoon of powdered enzymes and fresh acidophilus into this drink for maximum digestion perfection

See recipe #64 for directions on how to open up a young baby coconut.

Prep Time10m: | Serving: 2 | 100% Living

63. Good Morning Power Up Smoothie

Ingredients:

3	Bananas
3 cups	Pure Water
1/3 cup	Super Green Powder Blend*
1 tbsp.	Spirulina and Bee Pollen (each)
1 tbsp.	Honey
1 tbsp.	Powdered Vitamin C*
1 tbsp.	Liquid Chlorophyll
1 tbsp.	Powdered Enzymes*
2 tsp.	Powdered or liquid acidophilus
1/2 cup	Frozen or fresh blueberries (organic)

Directions:

Place all ingredients into blender and BLEND!

Jay's Tips:

This is Linda's favorite supergreen drink. If you do not get enough greens into your diet – this is a great substitute for those on the go, and still wanting to get their daily 'green fix'. *Our Supergreen Powders are a great addition but if you have your own, please make sure there are no sugars are additives in them.

Prep Time: 10m | Serving: 4 | 100% Living

64. The Date from Heaven Smoothie

Ingredients:

2	Young baby coconuts (use the meat & water)
2	Bananas
6	Dates
1/2 in.	Fresh ginger
1/3 cup	Macadamia nuts
1/3	Pineapple, peeled.
2 cups	Ice

Directions:

Blend all ingredients together and serve!

Linda's Tips:

Make sure to blend for a few minutes to make sure all ingredients are liquefied. We use a professional blender at home, and find it to be priceless and use it more than once per day. If you don't have a pineapple, you may substitute for two oranges. This is a fantastic drink for digestion troubled people. Young coconuts have a tremendous quality in them that helps heal the lining of the stomach, and combined with the fresh ginger, it doubles the healing power of this recipe.

How to open a Baby Coconut:

Young baby coconuts are a bit hard to open. We suggest using a very large knife (like a cleaver) - take it outside and cut off about 2 inches off the top, until you see part of the white meat showing. Take your finger and poke through the white meat whereby you will find the water. Save the water in a glass (it's very rich in minerals). Then take your cleaver and cut the coconut in half. From there it's very easy to scoop out the meat, and you can do so with a tablespoon.

Prep Time: 10m | Serving: 2 | 100% Living

65. Very Berry Powerful

Ingredients:

6-8	Apples (red or golden delicious)
6	Fresh Blackberries
6	Fresh Raspberries
1/2	Lime with skin
2	Oranges, peeled, retaining white pith
8	Fresh Blueberries
6	Strawberries

Directions:

Juice berries first, then follow through with apples, lime and orange.

Jay's Tips:

This is my personal favorite juice tonic for mornings. Remember, these berries are filled with powerful blood detoxifiers and brain stimulators. Best used only in the summertime when berries are fresh. If you want to use all year round, purchase organic berries frozen. Juice apples, then put all the rest of the ingredients in this recipe into the blender. Add one cup ice, and you have a wonderful smoothie.

Linda likes to add ice and one large, ripe banana to this recipe when she feels like a smoothie. Or, if you have frozen bananas in the freezer, that's a good substitute too. Hey, with smoothies costing close to $6.00 each, we make our own at home!

Jay's Juice Therapy Recipes

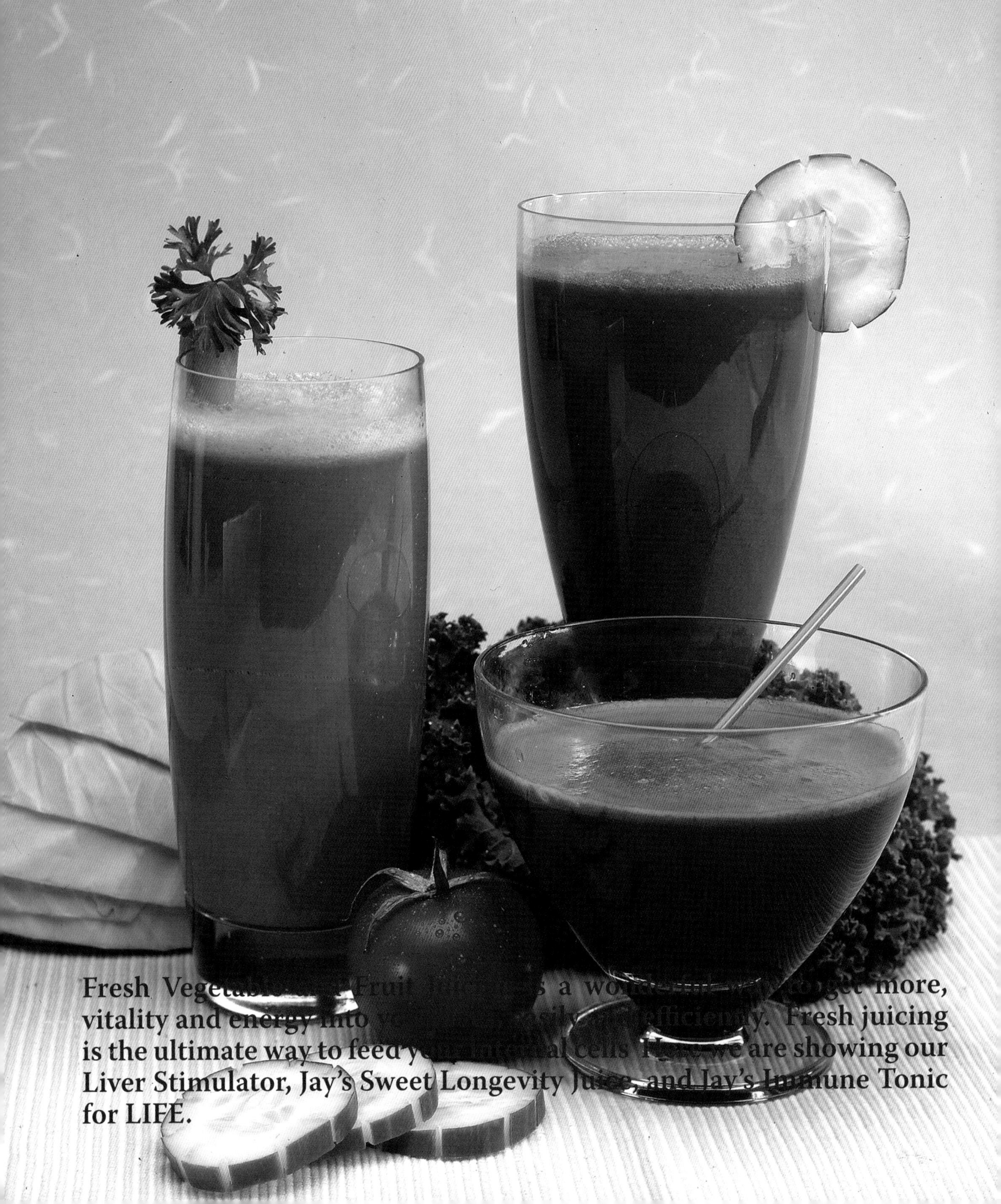

Fresh Vegetable and Fruit Juices is a wonderful way to get more, vitality and energy into your body easily and efficiently. Fresh juicing is the ultimate way to feed your internal cells. Here we are showing our Liver Stimulator, Jay's Sweet Longevity Juice, and Jay's Immune Tonic for LIFE.

Prep Time: 5m | Serving: 2 | 100% Living

66. Jay's Immune Tonic for LIFE

Ingredients:

10 Carrots
1 clove Garlic
1/2 Small beet with greens
1/2 Turnip
Handful purslane (ask your grocer)
Handful of spinach
Handful of kale (green or red)

Directions:

Juice greens first, then use the beet, then garlic, then finish with the carrots.

Jay's Tips:

Purslane is the key ingredient here. Try to find it-it's worth it. If you have the flu or a cold, this is my choice for a remedy. I try to drink over one quart per day to clean my system out.

Do not let your green juice set too long-it looses its enzyme properties and green power through oxidation

Prep Time:5m | Serving:2 | 100% Living

67. Enzyme-Rich Extravaganza

Ingredients:

2	Valencia Oranges, peeled with white peel left on as much as possible
2 inch	Pineapple, sliced lengthwise, peeled
2	Golden Delicious apples, quartered
1/2	Small papaya, skinned.
1/2 inch	Fresh organic ginger (peeled to avoid any fungus)

Directions:

Cut orange into juicer sized wedges. In the juicer, juice orange and pineapple, and ginger. Finish with the apple. In blender, blend the papaya and add the rest of the juice. Or you may juice the papaya along with all the other fruits. We prefer blending fruits such as papaya, as they are 99% water.

Jay's Tips:

Fantastic juice combination in the morning to get your digestion going. Great digestive aid. Do not drink this combination with a vegetable meal. Must either be consumed alone or with fruit salad.

Prep Time:5m | Serving: 2 | 100% Living

68. Jay's Sweet Longevity Juice

Ingredients:

1 cup	Riber (blackish purple) grapes
1 cup	Blackberries, raspberries or blueberries
1/2 inch	Fresh ginger root
1	Small lemon or lime
1	Green apple

Directions:

Juice all ingredients, using the apple last. This is a wonderful brain drink and energy drink also. If you are in spring/summertimes, add some ice to this drink. Or place one cup of ice into a blender and put juice inside blender, blend and there you've got a great smoothie, without any pulp.

Jay's Tips:

If you want to use this more as a smoothie, you can add a banana and put the juice into a blender with 1/2 cup ice. The Riber grapes are the key here. Because they have not been too hybridized, these grapes have very powerful immune building properties in them, thus the need to use these grapes only. Otherwise, if you cannot find them, use seeded red grapes, the darker the better.

69. Jay's Anti-aging Juice Tonic

Ingredients:

12	Carrots
1/2 cup	Wheatgrass
1/2 cup	Alfalfa greens
1/2 cup	Dandelion greens
3	Green apples
1 cup	Spinach
1/2	Medium sized Beet

Directions:

Juice wheatgrass first, then follow with 1/2 carrots. Then juice the greens next, followed through with the apples and rest of the carrots.

Jay's Tips:

This is a very green drink, but truthfully the best anti aging tonic I've been juicing since the 40's. Remember, when you're green inside, you're clean inside....and healthy!

Prep Time: 5m | Serving: 2 | 100% Living

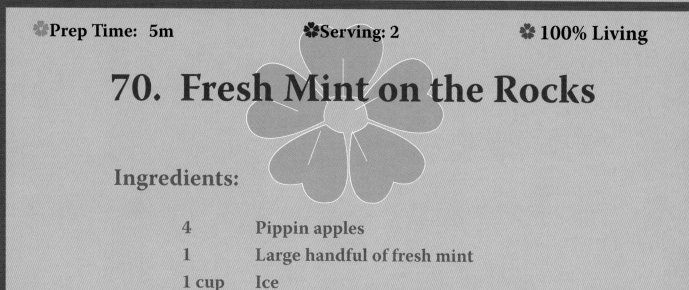

70. Fresh Mint on the Rocks

Ingredients:

4	Pippin apples
1	Large handful of fresh mint
1 cup	Ice

Directions:

In your juicer, juice the mint first, then flush through with all the apples. Strain the juice through a strainer, as to not allow the foam from the apples coat the ice.

Another version: When juice is finished, put the juice and ice into a blender and blend until smooth.

Put ice into a large glass-fill up the glass with the juice.

Jay's Tips:

Fabulous summertime for feeling overheated or over-exhausted.

✿Prep Time: 5m ✿ Serving: 2 ✿ 100% Living

71. Wheatgrass for Lightweights

Ingredients:

4	Organic Apples, any kind
2	Handfuls of Wheatgrass

Directions:

You must have a strong juicer to cut through and juice properly the wheatgrass.
Start off with the wheatgrass and juice 1/2 of the recipe first, then follow with 2 apples.
Repeat the above

Jay's Tips:

Do not store this particular juice combination. The powerful healing properties that lay inside wheatgrass dissipate very fast. Fantastic juice combination for stomach ailments.

Prep Time:5m   Serving:2   100% Living

72. My 3 "C's" Ulcer Tonic

Ingredients:

1/2	Green Cabbage
8	Carrots
4	Celery Stalks

Directions:

Cut the cabbage into long strips. Juice cabbage first, then follow with the celery stalks, then finish with the carrots.

Jay's Tips:

When I worked with Dr. Garnet Chaney back in the 1950's, we worked with ulcer patients using cabbage juice as a test. Over 90% of the patients lost their symptoms within 30 days, but they burped a lot! So we devised a way by adding celery and carrots to the recipe, which, when tested again, we found that we had the same results, and this time without any burping effects afterwards!

Prep Time: 5m | Serving: 2 | 100% Living

73. Pancreas Juice Happy Tonic

Ingredients:

10	Carrots
12	String beans
4	Brussels sprouts
2	Apples

Directions:

Start off first with juicing the string beans. Flush through with 5 carrots, then add all the brussels sprouts, then finish off with the apples and carrots to make sure all greens have been flushed through the juicer properly.

Jay's Tips:

This is a very strong tonic, and one that, used time and time again can really help build the pancreas into functioning better. Brussels sprouts and string beans make for a natural form of insulin, thereby helping the pancreas do its job better.

Prep Time: 5m | Serving: 2 | 100% Living

74. Jay's Vital Energy Tonic

Ingredients:

8	Carrots
1	Handful Spinach
1	Jerusalem artichoke
2	Apples
1	clove Garlic
2 inches	Fresh Burdock root

One handful parsley

Directions:

Juice 1/2 carrots with burdock root. Juice Jerusalem artichoke and greens next – then flush through with apples and the rest of the carrots

Jay's Tips:

This is a wonderful tonic for fast energy. If you are a woman, add 1/2 cup raw broccoli to this recipe for more energy and green power. This is not the best tasting tonic, but very powerfully energizing

Prep Time: 5m | Serving: 2 | 100% Living

75. Arthur-itis Helper

Ingredients:

3 inch	Fresh pineapple, peeled
1 inch	Fresh ginger root, peeled

Directions:

Cut the pineapple into strips that will fit through your juicer and juice with the ginger. You may want to add a golden delicious apple to flush out the pineapple, as it's a bit thick, and with the apple, it's easier to flush through.

Jay's Tips:

Fantastic juice combination for joint pain and good for aiding digestion.

Prep Time: 5m | Serving: 2 | 100% Living

76. Cucumber Cooler Healing Tonic

Ingredients:

1	Large Cucumber, peeled
1	Handful fresh mint
3	Large Apples, golden delicious

Directions:

Cut the cucumber in four pieces, starting with the cucumber, then add all the mint and use the apples to flush through the rest of the mint and cucumber from the bowl of the juicer as smaller greens have a tendency to stay in the bowl without a good flushing of the other fruits or vegetables.

Jay's Tips:

Great tonic for summertime by cooling the body. Also very good for reducing water retention in the body, and is a good excess body salt eliminator

Prep Time:5m **Serving: 2** **100% Living**

77. Positively in the PINK

Ingredients;

1	Pink Grapefruit, peeled-leaving as much white on the grapefruit as possible.
1 Cup	Fresh Raspberries
2	Red Delicious Apples, quartered

Directions:

Peel grapefruit. Place pieces into the juicer. In your juicer, juice grapefruit and finish with the apples. Pour juice into blender, add raspberries and blend till frothy. You may also use the raspberries in the juicer, but you won't be able to use 100% of them like you will with the blender.

Jay's Tips:

This is a fantastic tonic for your brain, and after exercising. I usually drink this tonic after I have a long workout or have been out in the sun for some time. This is when I add 1-2 cups ice during the summertime. Otherwise, it's fine just as it is, if it's during fall or wintertime.

Prep Time: 5m | Serving: 2 | 100% Living

78. Watermelon Kidney Whip

Ingredients:

2 Large slices cold watermelon

Directions:

Cut watermelon with the rind in approximately 2 inch pieces, or the size that fits through your juicer hole. Keep the rind only if it's an organic watermelon. If not organic, then soak in pesticide wash for 15 minutes beforehand.

Jay's Tips:

One of my favorite drinks in the summertime. Fantastic flushing effect on the kidneys. I usually eat watermelon, but when it's in season in the summertime, it makes for a wonderful drink. Only consume melons alone. Do not eat foods with watermelon or any melons. Also, I juice the watermelon with the skins because we only eat foods that are organic. You must only use the red part of the watermelon if you do not purchase your fruits organically. This is where juicing the entire watermelon comes in handy. A blender will not do this, nor I would not recommend eating the rind! It's very bitter. Just remember, organic!

Prep Time:5m | Serving: 2 | 100% Living

79. Liver Mover

Ingredients:

10 Medium Carrots

1 Beet, quartered

2 Apples, quartered

Directions:

Trim and cut carrots. In your juicer, juice carrots, alternating with beets and apples until all ingredients are juiced.

Jay's Tips:

This is a tonic my mentor, Dr. Gerson taught to me back in 1948. For anyone with a sluggish liver or an over-stimulated liver, this is a wonderful drink to consume on a daily basis. We love this tonic with a large vegetable salad such as recipe 11,12 or 13, located on page 124,125,126.

Prep Time:5m | Serving: 2 | 100% Living

80. Herby Goes Wild

Ingredients:

10	Medium Carrots
1	Handful fresh basil
1	Handful fresh parsley
2	Stalks Celery

Directions:

Trim and cut carrots. Bunch up basil and parsley tightly in your hands. Funnel through juicer, by pushing the carrots and celery through to get all the green juice through the bowl.

Jay's Tips:

This herbal living tonic is a fantastic drink for your liver and kidneys. Great with salads, spreads and semi-cooked foods.

Prep Time: 5m | Serving: 2 | 100% Living

81. V-12 Super Juice

Ingredients:

8-10	Medium Sized Carrots
1	Handful Parsley
1	Handful Cilantro
1/2	Red Bell Pepper
1	Large vine-ripened Tomato
1	Clove Garlic
1	Handful Spinach

Directions:

Start juicing with the greens, then flush through with the tomato, and finish off with the carrots.

Jay's Tips:

Rev your engines with this great V-12 juice drink. We love to use this tonic when eating mexican styled foods such as recipe # 88 and 90. Tofu Tacos, or Vegetarian Tacos located on page 210 and 212. It is especially nice after a workout.

Prep Time: 5m | Serving: 2 | 100% Living

82. Cranberry Kidney Surprise

Ingredients:

15-20	Fresh Cranberries
4-6	Golden Delicious apples

Directions:

Push cranberries through your juicer and finish with apples to make sure all cranberries have been properly flushed out of the bowl of the juicer.

Jay's Tips:

This is a great urogenital canal cleanser.

The fresh cranberries come out during the end of October and you can still purchase them through February. If you cannot find them fresh during the rest of the year, purchase extras for freezing. Then juice your apples, and blend the cranberries in the blender. Here's how you do it: Juice the apples, then put apple juice inside blender and put all the cranberries inside blender. Blend until liquefied. If you feel like it, try blending some ice cubes in this drink. If you have a fever or cold during wintertime, what a great way to get something cold down your throat, and have it be a healing tonic as well, with those powerful anti-oxidants in the cranberries.

Our Acceptable Cooked Food Recipes

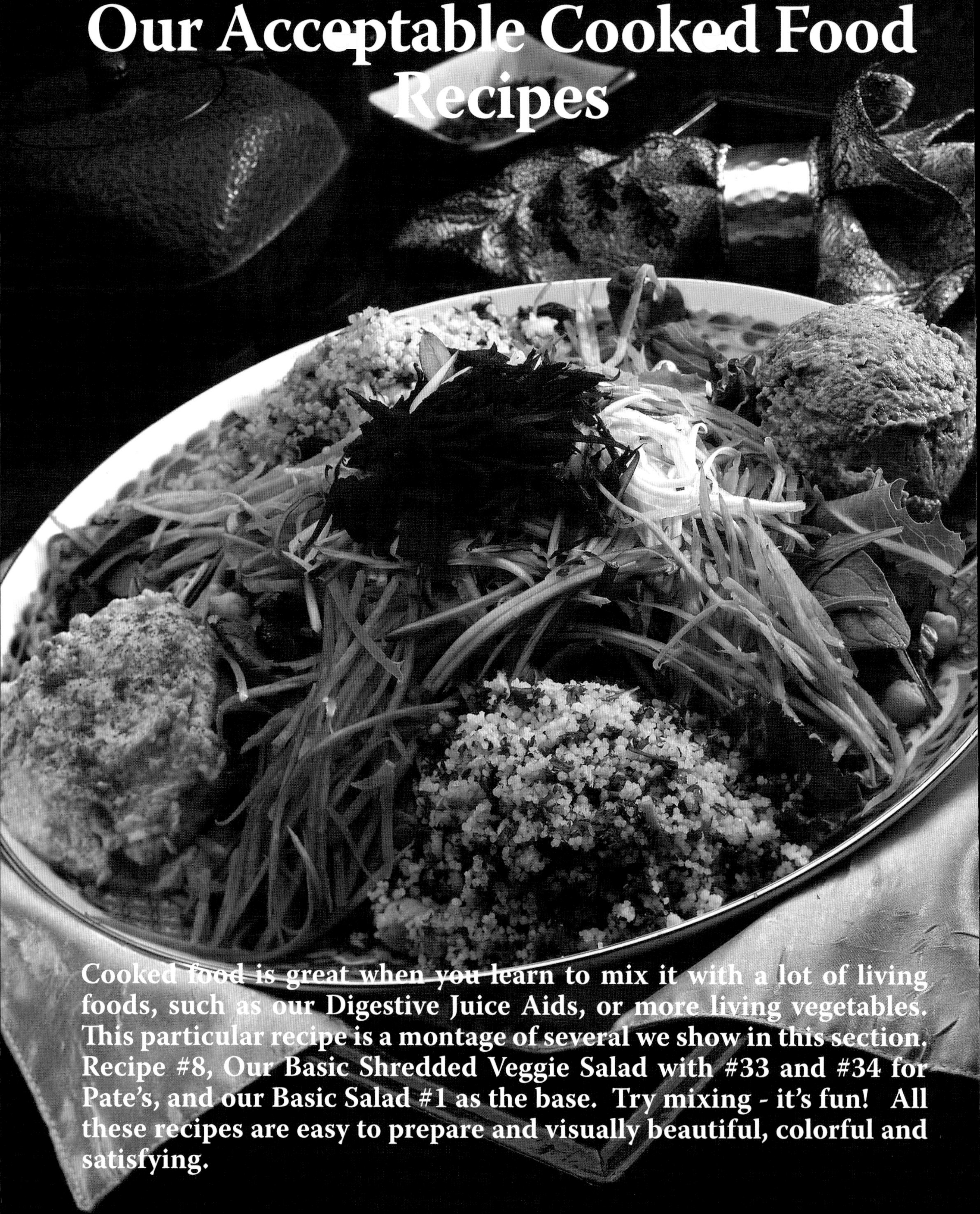

Cooked food is great when you learn to mix it with a lot of living foods, such as our Digestive Juice Aids, or more living vegetables. This particular recipe is a montage of several we show in this section. Recipe #8, Our Basic Shredded Veggie Salad with #33 and #34 for Pate's, and our Basic Salad #1 as the base. Try mixing - it's fun! All these recipes are easy to prepare and visually beautiful, colorful and satisfying.

Prep Time:15-20m | Serving: 4 | 80% cooked

83. Nutty Rice and Veggies

Ingredients:

4 cups	Short grain brown rice, cooked and hot.
2 tbsp.	Organic olive oil
3	Carrots, julienned
2	Stalks celery, chopped
1	Yellow or red bell pepper chopped
2 cups	Green onions, chopped
1 cup	Almonds, slivered
11/2 cup	Sunflower seeds
1/2 cup	Raisins
1 1/2 cups	(or 2 small) Haas Avocados, sliced (garnish)
1 large	Tomato, chopped (garnish)
1/2 cup	Black olives (pitted for garnish)
1/2 cup	Yellow onions, diced

Pepper to taste-either black or red

Directions:

In a serving bowl, combine all dried ingredients: almonds, sunflower seeds. Then add on top the bell pepper, onions, celery, carrots and raisins. Then add the very hot brown rice over all ingredients. Then add the oil. Keep in the oven for approximately 15 minutes. After it's had time to warm up the vegetables and other ingredients, bring out of the oven, toss and add the olive oil with the tamari.

Serve with all the garnished raw veggies on top. We recommend juice recipe # 72 , my 3 C's, located on page 193.

Linda's Tips:

Jay and I have eaten this recipe for over 20 years. We recommend putting as much living food on top of this recipe as possible. For example, you can add julienned yellow and green zucchini, sprouts (such as bean sprouts) more nuts, seeds and veggies, raw or steamed such as cauliflower. broccoli and/or our Asian Greens recipe #85 on page 207.

Prep Time: 15m | Serving: 4 | 100% Cooked

84. Carrot-Ginger Soup

Ingredients:

10	Carrots, diced or sliced thinly so it can cook faster
1inch	Fresh Ginger (peeled)
1	Medium sized Leek
12 cups	Pure water
1 1/2 tsp.	Nutmeg
1 tsp.	Sea salt
1/2 tsp.	Black pepper

Directions:

Cut all ingredients into small, one inch pieces. Slowly cook soup for approximately 20 minutes, or until carrots are soft. Blend in blender until desired consistency is achieved.

Linda's Tips:

Garnish with diced green onions, and or our salsa recipe #33 located on page 148 Great with one of our basic salads, such as our basic rice salad recipe #1 on page 113. and digestive juice aid #8 on page 21..

Prep Time: 15m | Serving: 4 | 100% Cooked

85. Asian Green Beans

Ingredients:

2 cups	Fresh organic green beans
1 tbsp.	Organic olive oil
1 tsp.	Dark, unrefined sesame oil
2 cloves	Fresh garlic, crushed
1 inch	Piece fresh ginger root, finely chopped
2 tbsp.	Nama shoyu or Tamari sauce

Directions:

Cut green beans diagonally. Steam in a stainless steamer or bamboo steamer the beans, until they turn darker green, and al dente (crisp to the touch). Meanwhile, in a sauce pan, add the oils (sesame and olive), then add the crushed garlic and ginger root. Cook only slightly until aroma starts to come up. Immediately add the nama shoyu or tamari, until the liquid has reduced, then pour over the warm beans.

Linda's Tips:

Recipe #20, Millet Basil Salad, on page 133 is a good match for these green beans. Just place the beans over the top of the Millet Salad and you have a whole meal salad. We also recommend Digestive Juice Recipe #10, on page 21 to go with this meal.

Prep Time:10m | Serving: 4 | 50-60% Living

86. Perfect Pita Sandwich

Ingredients:

2 cups	Romaine Lettuce, chopped
2	Tomatoes, chopped
1	Carrot, julienned
1	Zucchini, julienned
3	Green onions, chopped
1	Ripe Haas avocado, mashed
4	Whole grain Pita bread pockets
2 cups	Homemade Hummus -

(Recipe #36 on page 151)

Directions:

Stuff this pita pocket first with the hummus recipe. Then add in the following: avocado, zucchini, carrots, romaine lettuce, then the tomatoes, and then another dollop of hummus dressing, or you can substitute for dressing 37, Tomato Tofu Dressing on page 153.

Linda's Tips:

This is basically the only cooked bread we recommend, as it does not have yeast in the bread. Yeast is a toxic substance in breads (our opinion) and causes many digestive troubles, constipation and fungus. (kids love this recipe too.)

We recommend recipe # 22 on page 135, Jay's Favorite Beet Apple Salad, and recipe #6 on page 21 of our Digestive Juice Aids.

Prep Time: 15m | Serving: 4-6 | 100% Living

87. Our Lentil Burgers

Ingredients:

2	Stalks celery, diced
1/2	Medium onion, diced
1/2 cup	Parsley, diced
2	Clove garlic, crushed
1 1/2 cups	Rolled oats, uncooked
1/2 cup	Dried bread crumbs
1/2 cup	Pinto beans, cooked and mashed
1 cup	Lentils, cooked
1 tbsp.	Almond butter
1 tbsp.	Nama shoyu or Tamari

Sea salt and black pepper to taste.

Directions:

Dice celery, parsley, onion and garlic. In a mixing bowl, combine this mixture with remaining ingredients and mix well. Oil hands and form mixture into patties. In the oven, bake burgers until golden brown on top for 20 minutes each per side at 350 degrees.

Linda's Tips:

After trying for many years of experimenting is the best veggie-burger recipe we have created. Don't fret if they look strange in the beginning. When they are done, with browned tops, twenty minutes on each side in the oven, they look much better, and taste better than they look.

Garnish with as much living food as possible: tomatoes, onions, lettuce, sprouts, shredded veggies, stuffed inside a yeast free millet burger bun or some other yeast-free bun. Try recipe #44 on page 160, our "Superfast Tahini Dressing" or dressed over the top for a really moist yet tasty veggie-burger! Since this is mostly cooked, we recommend Digestive Juice Remedy #3, located on page 20

Prep Time: 15m | Serving: 4 | 50-75 % Living

88. Vegetarian Tacos

Ingredients:

8	Corn Tortillas
1 cup	Millet
4 tbsps.	Tamari or Nama Shoyu
2	Large ripe Haas avocados
1 cup (each)	Onion and organic olives, diced
1 cup	Romaine lettuce, chopped
1 cup	Tomatoes, chopped
1 cup	Zucchini – julienned or grated
1 cup	Carrots – julienned or grated
1 jar	Our Fresh Salsa (on page 148, recipe #33)

Directions:

Cook millet in 1 3/4 cups water to cover until done, about 30 minutes. Keep lid covered while cooking or else the millet gets dry. Meanwhile, prepare other ingredients. When millet is done, add the tamari or nama shoyu, mashed avocado, onions and mix well together. Heat tortillas in toaster oven or in a dry pan, or on gas burner (be careful). Then, place equal portions of millet mixture inside of the tortillas, top with lettuce, carrots, zucchini, and tomatoes. Finally, top with salsa.

Linda's Tips:

I personally love to put my humus #36, page 151 or #44 on page 160, (our superfast tahini dressing) over the top to make it taste moist and rich. This recipe is especially good for people allergic to common grains. We recommend Digestive Juice Aid #2 on page 20.

Prep Time:10m | Serving: 2-4 | 100% Cooked

89. Super easy Broccoli Soup

Ingredients:

3 cups	Broccoli, with stems
2 cups	Purified water
1	Vegetable bullion cube
1/2	Cup raw cashews

Seasalt, cayenne and black pepper to taste

Note: you may not need it because of the bullion cube, so wait until it's almost done before you add any more condiments.

Directions:

Put Broccoli inside pan with 2 1/2 cups water and bullion cube at the bottom. (make sure it doesn't get boiled, but lightly steamed).
3. When broccoli is ready, add all ingredients into blender.
Blend all ingredients together until you have reached the desired consistency. This soup is best when consumed within 24 hours. It does not store well.

Linda's Tips:

This recipe is so EASY! Great for lovers of 'cream of broccoli' that cannot tolerate dairy products. This soup is very filling. We suggest our Basic Salad Recipe #1 located on page 113 to go with this soup. Also, we recommend Digestive Juice Aid #1 on page 20.

Prep Time:10m | Serving: 4 | 75% Living

90. Tofu Tacos

Ingredients:

12 ounces	Firm Organic tofu
2 tbsps	Nama shoyu or soy sauce
1 tbsp	Lime juice
1 tbsp	Chili powder
1 tsp	Ground cumin
1 tsp	Garlic powder
1/4 tsp	Cayenne
3 cups	Shredded cabbage
2 cups	Julienne zucchini
8	Corn tortillas
1 cup	Salsa (recipe # 33 on page 148)
1 cup	Chopped tomatoes
1/4 cup	Chopped green onions

Directions:

Rinse tofu, drain in a colander for about 5 minutes, then pat dry with paper towels. Cut into 1-inch cubes and lightly blot with more paper towels. (Important). Bake the tofu in an oven at 400 degrees for 20 mins to brown and absorb flavors. In a bowl, mix soy sauce, lime juice, chili powder, cumin, crushed garlic, and cayenne. Add tofu and mix gently to coat cubes completely. Let stand 5 mins apprx. Take shredded cabbage, green narrowly sliced zucchini, chopped green onions, alfalfa sprouts, and mix in a bowl, together. Put the tortillas into the oven for about 5 mins to warm up and soften so you can put the ingredients into them without the tortilla splitting. Stack the tortillas with tofu first, then add the veggie mixture, then add the salsa on top.

Linda's Tips:

Adding Hummus #36, page 151 on the bottom of tacos would add a richer flavor. Digestive Juice Aid # 12 on page 21 is a good addition too, as it has cabbage in the juice recipe also.

✽ Prep Time: 10m ✽Serving: 4-6 ✽ 100% Cooked

91. Miso Healing Soup

Ingredients:

12 cups	Purified water
1	Foot strip of kombu seaweed
1/2 cup	Slivered carrots
3 cups	Chinese greens such as: Chinese Cabbage or Napa Cabbage.
2 cups	Organic watercress
1 cup	Chopped green onions (garnish)
1 cup	Sliced fresh oyster mushrooms
1 1/2	Cups dark miso
1 lb.	Block tofu, (soft), cubed

Directions:

Bring first two ingredients to a boil. Cut entire strip of kombu into long julienned strips. Begin adding other ingredients to water in the order listed. Hardest veggies go in first since they will take longer to cook. Place miso inside a fine screened strainer. Immerse bottom part of strainer into boiling water and mash miso through the screen into the water with the back of a large spoon. This makes a smoother soup. Add cubes of tofu and cook long enough to warm. Serve with our flax crackers located on page 172, recipe #54.

Linda's Tips:

Great soup when you are feeling emotional, needing a little TLC. This soup with give you a lot of comfort. The kombu adds wonderful minerals and essential vitamins to this soup. We suggest a simple salad such as Our Basic Salad #1 and #1a for the dressing.

In wintertime, it's good to add long grain brown rice to this dish. (I just put it in the middle of the miso soup), then add raw green onions on top.

Prep Time: 15m | Serving: 4 | 50-75% Living

92. It's a Whole World Tostada

Ingredients:

4	Spinach tortillas
1 cup	Romaine Lettuce, chopped
1 cup	Shredded green cabbage
1 cup	Grated or julienned carrots
1 cup	Julienned green zucchini
1/2 cup	Olives, diced or sliced
1/2 cup	Onions, diced
1 cup	(salsa on page 148, recipe #33)
1/2 cup	Each cilantro and parsley
2 1/2 cups	Cooked black beans
1 cup	Super simple guacamole (page 146, recipe #31)

Directions:

Heat Beans and keep on stove until ready to put together your tostada. Shred, chop, grate or julienne the following: zucchini, carrots, onions, cilantro, parsley, tomatoes, cabbage and olives

Prepare our simple guacamole (recipe # 31 on page 146) and keep in the refrigerator. Prepare salsa at the same time as our simple guacamole for the recipe

Heat tortillas on the stove in a pan without any oil until they start to bubble and heat up to be able to withstand enough weight to build your tostada. Keep your eye on the pan at all times, as they can heat up very fast. We use two tortillas instead of one to make for a thicker tostada base.

Prep Time:15m | Serving: 4 | 50-75% Living

Whole World Tostada, pt.2

Directions, continued:

Once your tortillas are heated up, place in order the following:

1. Black beans
2. Onions
3. Romaine lettuce and cabbage
4. Carrots and zucchini
5. Cilantro and parsley
6. Guacamole and olives
7. Salsa and tomatoes

Linda's Tips:

We love this recipe and it is very, very easy to prepare. Don't let all the ingredients intimidate you. If you only have cabbage or just romaine, just use that, but with all the ingredients together, it's great. It makes an entire meal for the family. Jay and I recommend drinking Digestive Juice Recipe #4, page 20 with this visually beautiful meal.

Prep Time:15m | Serving: 4 | 75% Cooked

93. Veggie Wrap

Ingredients:

2	Large red potatoes, cooked and cubed
3	Carrots, julienned
1 small	Cauliflower, chopped into flowerets
2 cups	Short grain brown rice (cooked)
2 cup	Black bans, cooked
2 cups	Thai peanut Sauce (page #94)
2 cups	Romaine lettuce, chopped
1 cup	Alfalfa or sunflower sprouts
1 cup	Fresh cilantro
1 large	Clove garlic, crushed
4	Burrito style Spinach or Basil tortillas

Directions:

In a steamer, steam potatoes for 10 to 15 minutes, then add carrots and cauliflower for another few minutes. Cover and allow to sit for another five minutes. In a large mixing bowl, combine vegetables with rice, beans and our peanut sauce and mix well. In a skillet on medium heat, warm a tortilla until it is soft and pliable. Spread with vegetable and rice mixture, then lettuce and sprouts and cilantro. Roll up while tucking in the ends and place on plate seam side down. You may want to cover over the top with more dressing.

Linda's Tips:

Because of the peanuts, this is a heavy recipe, so we recommend highly you use a Digestive Juice Aid # 4 on page 20. If you cannot drink juice or don't have time to make it, then we recommend you sprinkle fresh raw onions inside of the wrapped Buddha.

Prep Time: 15m | Serving: 4 | 100% Living

94. Veggie Wrap Sauce
(Thai peanut dressing)

Ingredients:

1/4	fresh lime juice
3 Tbsp.	Creamy (un-hydrogenated) peanut butter and not roasted
3 tbsp.	Tamari
3 tbsp.	Honey
2 tbsp.	Chili paste
4 cloves	garlic, minced

Directions:

Combine all ingredients in a blender and blend until desired consistency is achieved. Makes 1/2 cup

Linda's Tips:

This is a great dressing/sauce/dip. As you can see it's versatile and tastes great. I suggest using this over any wrap you create. It's also very good over recipe #85, Asian Green Beans on page 207, or drizzled over any of our living soups for a richer taste.

~Make your own Recipe~

~Make your own Recipe~

~Make your own Recipe~

~Make your own Recipe~

~Make your own Recipe~

~Make your own Recipe~

~Make your own Recipe~

~Make your own Recipe~

“You Always have
Change At This M

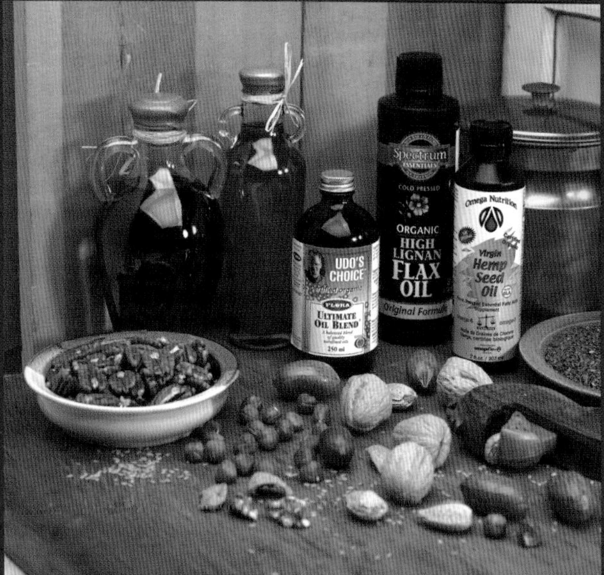

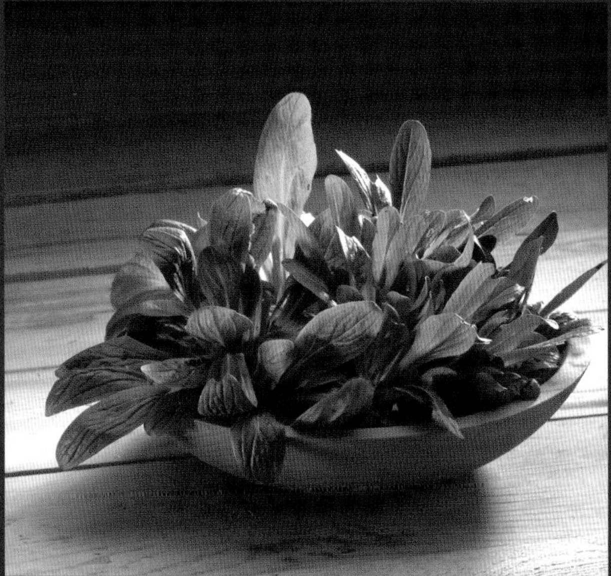

the Power to
oment" *Jay Kordich*

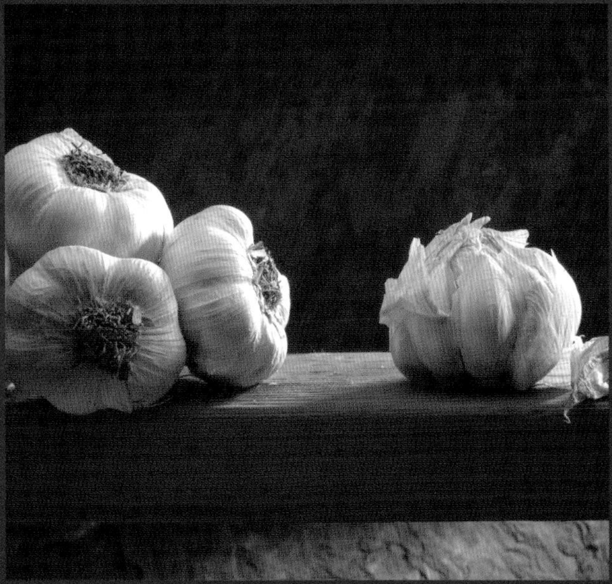

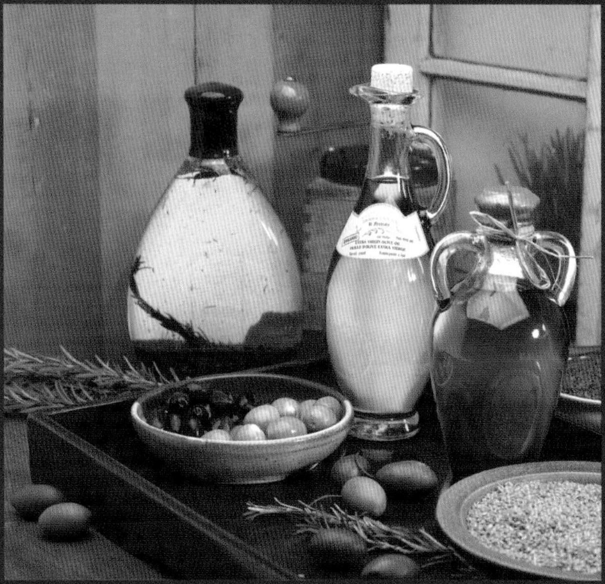

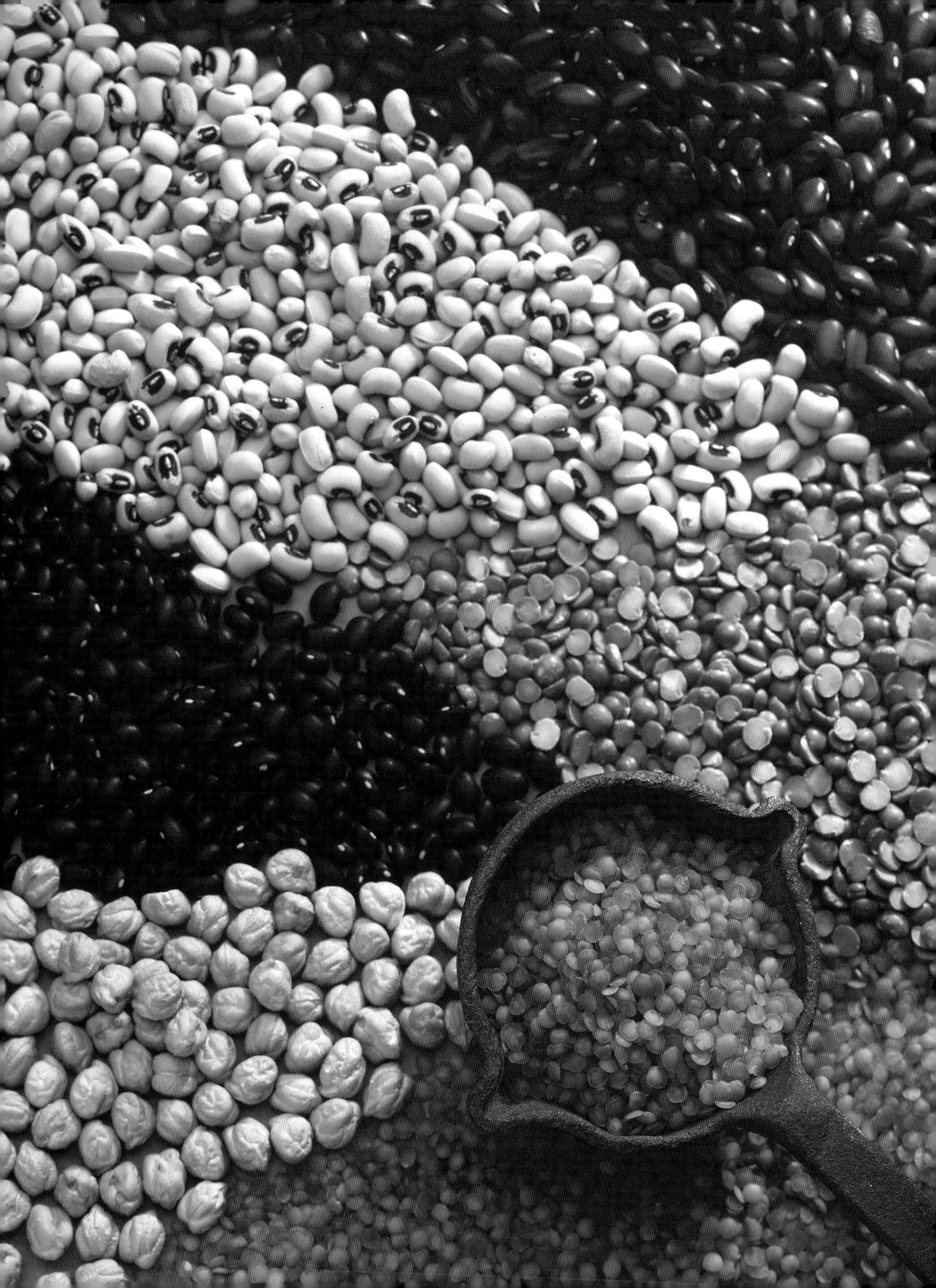

Our Personal Web site & Resources

In this final section of our book, we would to share our personal resources with you.

Throughout the years, while we have been working on this book, teaching seminars on juicing and living foods, we have accumulated a list of reliable and knowledgeable resources and web sites that we highly recommend.

We believe, that as you start to transition towards a better diet, you will need all the support possible without falling prey to hype and fluff that can steer you in the wrong direction. Because your vital health depends on the right resources, we want to make sure you are going in the right direction. We hope you will find this section of our book useful and supportive.

SPROUTS

The Sprout People
www.sproutpeople.com
Wide selection of sprouts and seeds for home sprouting. Mail order available.
225 Main Street
Gays Mills, WI 54631
608 735 4735 phone/fax

HERBS

American Botanical Council
www.herbalgram.org
Publishes the journal Herbalgram, available for a fee. Write for catalog
P.O. box 302660
Austin, TX 78720
512 331 8868

The American Herbalists Guild
www.americanherbalistsguild.com
Offers a directory of herbal education
P.O. box 1683
Soquel, CA 95073

Herb Research Foundation
www.herbs.org/herbs
1007 Pearl St #200 F
Boulder Co 80302

Smokey Santillo-author
Food Enzymes, the Missing Link to Radiant Health

HEALTH PRACTITIONERS

Dr. Vincent Savarese (chiropractor)
10447 Magnolia Blvd.
North Hollywood, California
(818) 769 1811
72724 29 Palms Hwy.
29 Palms, California
(760) 361-0087

The Flower Essence Society
www.flowersociety.org

The Society was founded by Richard Katz in 1989. 72 or more flower-based remedies have been discovered and used for emotional challenges. I highly recommend getting on their site.
Box 459
Nevada City, CA 95959
916-265 9163

Lightkin Shen Therapy and Personal Flower Essence Remedies.
Ayleyaell Kinder
(619) 584-1077

Blessed Herbs
www.blessedherbs.com

great organic fresh or dried herbs you can order via mail order or online
109 Barre Plains Road
Coahoma, MA 01063

BOOKS ON HERBS
Back to Eden-Jethro Kloss
The tell all be all herbal book that is over 75 years old

JUICE THERAPY
A Cancer Therapy: Results of Fifty Cases and their Cures
Advanced Cancer Diet Therapy
by Dr. Max Gerson, M.D.
Station Hill Press, 1990

The Juiceman's Power of Juicing
by Jay Kordich
William Morrow, 1992

The Complete Book of Juicing
By Michael T Murray, N.D.
Prima Publishing, 1992

LIVING FOOD ORGANIZATIONS:

Tree Of Life Rejuvenation
Dr. Gabriel Cousins
www.treeoflife.nu
Medical/Psychiatrist Dr.,Natuopathic Doctor and esteemed author on living foods.

Ann Wigmore Foundation
www.wigmore.org
The birthplace of wheatgrass and live foods training. Programs
Available world-wide. Formerly known as Hippocrates Health Institute
P.O. box 140
Toreon, NM 87061

Gerson Institute
www.gerson.org
The original raw juice therapy program Jay Kordich went on and driven now
By Dr. Gerson's daughter, Charlotte Gerson Strauss. Live-in alternative therapy treatment center and cancer clinic on location
P.O. Box 430
Bonita, CA 9l908
619 267 1150

Optimum Health Institute
www.optimumhealth.org
free classes, clinics, spa and lectures
live-in school of nutrition, centered on detoxification and wheatgrass
therapy
6970 Central Avenue
Lemon Grove, CA 91945 619 464 3346

ORGANIC FOOD ORGANIZATIONS:

*California Certified Organic Farmers
www.ccof.org
Promotes organic agriculture and certifies organic growers
And processors in California. A list of local organic growers listed.

ORGANIC FOOD SOURCES

Bates Nut Farm
(no web site yet, but worth ordering via mail order)
15954 Woods Valley Road
Valley Center, CA 92082
760 749 3333
800 642 0348

Fiddler's Green Farm
www.fiddlersgreenfarm.com
A certified organic family farm producing freshly stone-ground flours
Jams and other foods. Free mail order catalog.
Belfast, ME 04915
800-729-7935
207 338 3568

Gem Cultures
www.gemcultures.com
Offers fermented foods like cabbage, tempeh, miso. Also carries
Bulk items.
30301 Sherwood Road
Fort Bragg, CA 95437
707 964 2922

*Seeds of Change
www.seedsofchange.com
Seller of only certified organic, open pollinated seeds for backyard gardeners.

Large selection of heirloom and traditional varieties of vegetable, herbs and flower seeds. Catalog available.
621 Old Santa Fe Train, #10
Santa Fe, NM 87501
505 983 8956

SPROUTING ORGANIZATIONS

Gourmet Greens
www.gourmetgreens.com
Specializes in soil grown sprouts and fresh wheatgrass
RR#4, Box 560B
Chester, VT 05143
802 875 3820

MAGAZINES

Natural health Magazine
www.naturalhealthmagazine.com
Articles on all aspects of well-being
Through natural methods and healing foods

Eating Well
www.eatingwell.com
Each month specializes on one particular food in season.
One of our favorite magazines-hardly any adds.

Vegetarian Times
www.vegetariantimes.com
The leader in the vegetarian movement since mid 1970's.
Great articles on foods, lifestyle and recent research

SUPPORT GROUPS AND ORGANIZATIONS
These organizations provide excellent support for the new or curious

Vegetarian or non-vegetarian. You can order books, get recipe ideas or network together either online or through meeting
American Vegan Society
www.americanvegan.org
p.o. box H
Malaga, NJ 8328
609 694 2288

Earth Save
www.earthsave.org
706 Frederick Street
Santa Cruz, CA 95062
408 423 0255
Sponsors the Health School Lunch program. Call for information about good foods served in your school cafeteria, including a comprehensive action handbook of students, parents and teachers

PRODUCTS FOR ORDERING

Ahler's Organic Date and Grapefruit Garden
www.localharvest.org
P.o. Box 726
Mecca, CA 92254

Dr. Bronner's Products
www.drbronner.com
Dr. Bronner's barleymalt sweeteners, liquid castile soaps (homemade)
Balanced mineral bouillon cubes and seasonings, and many other items.
One of our favorite sites
Box 28
Escondido, CA 92025

Omega Life, Inc.
www.brightspot.org
flaxseed, ground to powder and combined with nutritional co-factors
15355 Woodbidge Road

Brookfield, WI 53005

Thistle Dew Farms
www.thistledewfarm.com
fine gifts from the honeybee including honeycomb, honey, honey mustard, beeswax, skin cream and candle. Mail order available.
304 455-1728 ph
304 455 1740 fx
005
800 328 3529

Frontier Cooperative Herbs
www.frontiercoop.com
Many herbs and other natural products for sale
Box 69
Norway, IA 52318

Spring Tree Corporation
www.springtree.com
Mail Order also – organic maple syrup and carob powder
P.O. Box 1160
Brattleboro, VT 05301
802 254-8784

*Beck Grove
www.localharvest.org
many varieties of fruits. Specializes in kumquats, blood oranges, fuyu persimmons, Satsuma mandarin oranges and Minneola's.
Mail order available also.
P.O. box 2890
Fallbrook, CA 9288
760 728 9007

Blue Heron Botanicals
www.localharvest.org
154 Van Duzen River road
Bidgeville, CA 95526
707 574 6574

Blue Heron Farm
www.wintercreekgardens.com
p.o. box 68
Rumsey, CA 95679
916 796 3799

Cherry Moon Farms
www.cherrymoonfarms.com
Wonderful organic and non organic foods online for delivery anywhere in the U.S. (gift oriented)
1-888-378 2758

Sun Organic Farms
www.sunorganicfarm.com
Organic Foods galore, and a wonderful web site. We love this company.
1888 269 9888

Four Apostles Ranch
www.fourapostles.com
Organically grown unsulfured medjool dates.
Mail order available
760 345 6171

Frog Hollow Farm
www.froghollowfarm.com
Tree ripened peaches, nectarines, asian pears, cherries and able grapes
For delivery
510 634 2845
McFadden Farm
www.mcfaddenfarm.com
Organic Herbs fresh and dried, sundried tomatoes, beans and wine grapes
Mail order available as well as online
PotterValley, CA 95469

Mendocino Sea Vegetable company
www.seaweed.net
Wildcrafted, dried North America sea vegetables.
Mail Order Available.

*Rising Tide Sea Vegetables
www.loveseaweed.com
Harvest primarily Wakame, Kombu, Sea palm and Nori sea vegetables. Some sea vegetable condiments and snacks also.

*Live Food Organics
www.ilovekale.com
www.greencoconuts.com
Organic Baby Coconuts and superfoods, raw food snacks included.
We love this site, and order our young baby coconuts from this site when
They are not available at our local health food store.

*Noni Fruit Leather
Nonifruitleather.net
Located in Kauai, Hawaii owned by Steve Frailey
Only uses organic noni – wonderful company and great web site
808 585 9988

Puna Organics

Puna gold Hawaiian (Japanese) yellow ginger, mail order
Catalog available (no web site)
P.o. Box 3298
Pahoa, HI 96778
808 965 7088 Phone

Charan Springs Farm
www.organickitchen.com
wonderful organic salad mixes and greens, avocados, vegetables and sprouts. Check out their web site!
805 927 8287

Wood Prairie Farm
www.woodprairie.com
Organic seed and tablestock potatoes, speciality items, but generally
A great site for information and ordering online or via phone
4946 Kinney Road
Bridgewater, ME 04735
800 829 9765 ph
800 300 6494 fax

Wise Ways herbal/singing Brook Farm
www.mysticunicorn.com
Organic herbal products, bath crystals, salves, lip alms, oils, creams extracts, teas and hair and body care. All handmade and wildcrafted.

Ozark Forest Mushrooms
www.ozarkforest.com
Shiitake, Oyster and Pom Pom mushrooms Mail order available.
314 531 9935 ph/fax

Herb Pharm
www.herb-farm.com
full line of herbal extracts from organically and wildcrafted herbs. Mail order also available as well as online.
20260 Williams Highway
P.O. box 116
Williams, OR 97544
541 846 6261 ph
800 545 7392 fax

Homestead Organic Produce
www.organicexpress.com
Red and golden delicious apples, fuji and granny smith apples as well as Korean red hot garlic, storage onions and alfalfa for sale.
20034 Road 7 NW
Quincy, WA 98848
509 787 2248

South Tex Organics, LC
www.stxorganics.com
Citrus and vegetables specializing in organic Rio Star Grapefruit, early and late season oranges, carrots, potatoes, spring sweet yellow and red onions and watermelon
210 585 1040

Mineral Salts
www.saltworks.us
www.seasalt.com
We love both these sites, and are primarily online stores. This is where
We purchase our celtic sea-salts from home

ENZYMES
Kordich Group International
jaykordich.com
p.o. box 3486
Rancho Santa Fe, Ca. 92067

~*Personal Notes*~

~Personal Notes~

Index

A

acceptable foods 82
achy feeling 17
addicted 17
addiction 59
affirmation 85, 87
alcohol 50
all berries 12
almond milk 50, 79
Aluminum cookware 81
alzheimers disease 81
amylase 47
anger 17
animals 60
animal products 48
antiseptic 48
apple 20, 21
Apples 66
apples 85
appliances 5
Appreciation 104
arthritis 48
artificial colors 83
artificial sweeteners 83
art of salad making 100
assimilation 69
astringent 94
atoms 15
attention, 87
Automatic sprouter 82
awareness 81
ayurveda 94

B

balanced 47
banana 12
bananas 47
Barbecues 81
barley 50
beauty 79
Berries 66
berries 12, 61, 85
bitter 94
black tea 16
black tea. 16
bleeding ulcers 48
bloating 48
bloodstream 22
blossom 76
body-active 14
Boerner slicer 82
boils 17
bok choy 16
borage 83
boron. 15
bowels 22
brain 46
broccoli 16, 60
bromelain 47
broths 12
Brown rice 62
Brussels Sprouts 13
Brussels sprouts 13
budget 82
Bulghur 62

C

cabbage 21
Caffeine 50
caffeine 60
caffix 50
cakes, 83
calcium 15
calcium propionate, 83
cancer 7
cancerous cells 47

candy bars 83
canned foods 82
cantaloupe 12
carbonated drinks 50
carrot 47
carrots 20, 21
catalyst 49
cathartic 15
cauliflower 60
celery 20, 21
cellular 75
cellular level 48
cellular walls 15
chamomile 16
chemotherapy 11
cherries 61
Chew 51
chewing 49
chips, 83
cilantro 85
cobalt 11
coffee 50, 58
Coffees 83
coffee creamers, 83
Coffee maker 81
coffee substitutes 50
cola 50
cold press 69
colitis 47, 48
colon 48
colonics 98
colon cleanse 46
colored vegetables 77
constipation 48
contemplation 15
cooked grains 94
cookies, 83
Copper cookware 81
Cosmic Energy Principle 46
cottonseed oils, 83
creativity. 76
Crisco, 83
crushed garlic 48
cucumber 21
cucumbers 22

D

de-stress. 100
dedication 81
Deep-fat fryers 81
Dehydrator 82
Deli meats 83
detoxification 17
devitalized foods 45
Diarrhea 17
Diet For a New America 91
digestive ailments 47
digestive juices 50
digestive troubles 48
discouraged 81
Dishes containing lead 81
Disorientation 17
dizziness 17
doctor 17
dough conditioners 83
Dr. Edward Howell 46
Dr. Gabriel Cousins 13
Dr. Gabriel Cousins, Spiritual Nutrition 46
Dr. Humberto Santillo 46
Dr. Norman Walker 13
Dr. Vince Savarese 229
dried herbs 79
dry body brush 15
dysfunctional 76

E

eating disorder 59
eBay 82
Electric tea pot 82
Electronic pesticide remover 82

elimination 14
emotional nourishment 59
empowered 76
endive 16
Enya 85
enzyme 45
enzyme-rich 84
enzymes 6, 46, 51
enzyme amylase 47
enzyme inhibitor 62
enzyme papain 47
esoteric 104
Europe 11
evolution 75
Evolution Organic Baby Field Greens. 85

F

fasting 12
Fear 46
flash-frozen 86
flax 83
Fletcherizer Method 51
Foods 57
food labels 82
Food processor 82
food shelter 82
foreign bacteria 48
fragrances 79
Fruitarian 67
fruits 59
frustration 17

G

Gabriel Cousins 46
gardening 76
gardens 76
garlic 48
ginger 16, 21
ginger. 16
Glass containers f 82
goal 58
God 99
grains 59
grandparents 76
grateful 87
greens 59
green beans 60, 61
Green juices 22
green tea 16
Grills aluminum or Teflon coated 81
grocery shopping 104

H

Habit 101
Hand-held blender 82
Headache 17
health practitioner. 17
hearts 75
hemp oil 71
herbal teas 79
Herbs 57
herbs 59
honey 50
honey. 50
honor 100
Humberto Santillo 46
hybridized 13
hydrogenated 83
hydrogenated oil- 79

I

Illness 12
infomercial 5
inhibitors 69
inorganic 15
insulin 13
Integration 98

intention 87
intestines 22
iron 15

J

Jay Kordich 57
John Robbins 91
Josh Groban 85
joyful 76
juice 16
juicers 5
juice bar 14
juicing 5, 14

K

Kailua, Hawaii 14
kale 16, 20, 21
ketchup 83
kidney stone 81
kiwi, 85
kiwis 12
knives, bowls, appliances, kitchen tools, herbs, and spices 80

L

lard 83
lavender oil 15
laxative 15
leaky gut 48
leaky gut syndrome 47
Linda 6
liver 22
Living Foodist 67
Living foods 6, 59
living health 81
love 87
lungs 45
l laxative 15

M

Macadamia nuts 71
magical 102
mango 12
margarine 83
Max Gerson 7, 11
mayonnaise 83
meat 14
meditation 15
melon 12
melons 12
metaphysical 81
Millet 62
minerals 13, 15
molecules 46
mono diglycerides, 83
Mother Nature 99
mucus 17
muffins 83
mushrooms 85
mustards 83
mustards, relishes, tomatoes, and egg-free mayonnaise, salsas and nut butters. 79
My Kitchen Sanctuary— 98

N

natural antiseptic 48
Nausea 17
nitrates 83
nitrites 83
Non-stick cookware 81
Norman Walker 13
Nuts 68
nuts 59
Nut and seed grinder 82
nut butters 83

O

Oats 62
Oils 69
Omega 3 69
Omega 6 69
onions 48, 79
Our Living Kitchen program. 80
oxidation 51
oxygen 22

P

packaged foods 82
Pancreas 13
pancreatic enzymes 47
pantries 79
papain 47
papaya 12, 47
parasitses 48
parsley 16, 20, 21, 85
partially hydrogenated oils 83
Partners 104
pasteurized 14
peaches 61, 85
peanut oil 83
Pearl barley 62
pears 61
peppermint 16
peristaltic wave 22
pero 50
pet. 87
philosophies 87
phosphorus, 15
photosynthesis 15
physical nourishment 59
phytochemicals 13
phytonutrients 6
pies 83
Pimples 17
pineapple 47
plant life 15
plums 85
pomegranates 61
potatoes 71, 79
power 102
prayer 15
predigested food 47
prisoner 100
processed foods 60, 79
Professional grade knives 82
professional juicer, high-powered blender, food processor, dehydrator, electric tea pot, steam distiller, bamboo steamer, and multi-grain rice cooker. 79
Pumpkinseed oil 70
pungent 94
purifying 22
putrifaction 14

Q

Quinoa 62

R

radiation 11
rancid. 83
raw 7
raw onions 48
Raw Vegetable Juicing 13
refrigerators 79
regenerates 48
relaxation 15
relaxing bath 15
religions 87
relish 83
reverse osmosis 50
rice milk 50
rice milk, 50
Rotisseries and/or Roasters 81
runny nose 17

S

safflower oils, 83
salads 71, 83
Salad spinner 82
salsas 83
sanctuary 100
sauerkraut 83
seasons 59, 60
seeds 59
simple diet 102
simplicity. 102
soak 69
Soaking 62
soft drinks 83
soil 14
soul 87
sour 94
Soymilk 50
Soymilk maker 82
sparkplug 15
Spices 57
spices 79
spinach 16, 20, 21, 85
spiritual 87
spiritual force, 99
Spiritual Nutrition 46
spring 60
sprouted seed 94
squashes 61
stainless steel wok 82
starches 48
steam-distilled 50
steaming 60
Steam distiller 82
stone fruits 12
storage 82
string beans 13
sugar 60
sugars 48
sulfur dioxide 83
summer 60
sun tea 82
superior digestion 13
Supreme Father 87

T

Tecchino 50
Teflon-coated cookware 81
Teflon-coated frying pans 81
terminally ill 48
thermos 51
The 75/25 Principle 57
The Power of Living Foods 5, 75
Tofu 83
Tofu maker 82
tomatoes 61, 85
tools 80
toxemia 46
trademark 12
trauma 59

U

unhealthy 76
University of Southern California 11
unpasteurized 83
unsweetened 86
urinary tract. 22
utensils 81

V

Vegan 67
vegetables 59
vegetable juicing 57
Vegetarian 67
Vegetarian foods 6
Vitality 45
Vince Savarese 229

W

walking 15
walnut oil 71
water 17
Weakness 17
wheatgrass 16
Wheatgrass juicer 82
wheat products 60
white bread 48
White flour 83
White rice 83
White sugar 83
whole meal salads 91
wine 83

Y

Yanni 85
yeast 83
yoga 15

Z

zinc 15